Jennifer Erin Camulli
Guo-Hui Xie

Tuberous Sclerosis Complex with Syndromic Autism

Jennifer Erin Camulli
Guo-Hui Xie

Tuberous Sclerosis Complex with Syndromic Autism

A Case review of an Autistic Savant Artist

LAP LAMBERT Academic Publishing

Imprint

Any brand names and product names mentioned in this book are subject to trademark, brand or patent protection and are trademarks or registered trademarks of their respective holders. The use of brand names, product names, common names, trade names, product descriptions etc. even without a particular marking in this work is in no way to be construed to mean that such names may be regarded as unrestricted in respect of trademark and brand protection legislation and could thus be used by anyone.

Cover image: www.ingimage.com

Publisher:
LAP LAMBERT Academic Publishing
is a trademark of
International Book Market Service Ltd., member of OmniScriptum Publishing Group
17 Meldrum Street, Beau Bassin 71504, Mauritius

Printed at: see last page
ISBN: 978-620-0-53937-3

TUBEROUS SCLEROSIS COMPLEX WITH SYNDROMIC AUTISM: A CASE REVIEW OF AN AUTISTIC SAVANT ARTIST

Jennifer Erin CAMULLI, PhD
Guo Hui Xie, EdD

ABSTRACT/BLURB

This is a case review of a young savant artist diagnosed with Tuberous Sclerosis Complex (or TSC for short). According to the Online Mendelian Inheritance in Man® (OMIM), there are two types of TSC, with two different code/classification numbers: (i) #191100 for TSC Type 1, and (ii) #613254 for TSC Type 2. Both TSC types have associated comorbidities such as autism, developmental delay and intellectual disability. The aim of this monograph is to provide diagnostic information about the syndrome with its comorbidities so that educational therapists and other allied professionals working with such individuals will know what to look for, especially the TSC-associated comorbidities, and in that way, they become better informed to know what to offer in their Response to Intervention (RtI) for such individuals with TSC.

Key words: Autism Spectrum Disorder, Savant Syndrome, Tuberous Sclerosis Complex

BRIEF BIODATA

Jennifer Erin CAMULLI, PhD: Studied education at the University of Victoria, British Columbia, Canada, and the University of Saint Joseph, Macau, PRC. IACT-certified special needs educational therapist and accessibility and inclusion consultant serving in Dubai, United Arab Emirates.

Guo-Hui XIE, EdD: Studied education at the University of Western Australia, Perth. Board-certified in educational therapy and special education. IACT-approved instructor. Special needs consultant serving in South-East Asian region.

CHAPTER ONE
A BRIEF INTRODUCTION TO A CASE OF TUBEROUS SCLEROSIS COMPLEX

Tuberous sclerosis complex (TSC) is one of several autosomal disorders that can manifest multiple symptoms ranging from mild to life-threatening. When more severe symptoms occur, other co-occurring conditions, or even talents, can be masked or harder to detect. Educational therapists and allied professionals may errantly attribute the symptoms to the primary disorder alone, such as TSC, and implement insufficient intervention or miss an opportunity to develop a talent, due to incomplete information of the individual.

A Brief Introduction to BK - the Man with Tuberous Sclerosis Complex

This monograph presents this case of a young Chinese man, BK[1], 31 years 1 month old at the time of this study, who had previously been diagnosed with tuberous sclerosis complex from a young age. The authors have known BK's family for the past three years through an educational therapist, who is a close friend of the family, and observed remarkable artistic skills that warranted further investigation. The authors met the young man and his family and viewed his art work and determined that psycho-educational assessment and profiling would help to determine if BK qualifies for the diagnosis of Savant Syndrome.

BK's Schooling History

As reported by Goh and Xie (2019), BK was enrolled in a kindergarten in May 1990. His mood was observed to be consistent and he was able to fit into the kindergarten. Within a few days, he was able to adapt well in the new environment. Unfortunately, he suffered a relapse of epileptic attack while in the kindergarten, and his preschool teachers described him as someone who "loses his head."

BK was noted by his preschool teachers to be a very closed-up child whose appearance and functional level were strongly characterized by his stereotyped behaviour. BK spent most of his time being "private" or sedentary. "However, there were times when he would dash about in class in a certain fixed pattern, make monotonous sounds with his mouth or with some objects, play (manipulate) with saliva either in his mouth or spat on the surface, and was very fixated by lines he could find and sun rays, etc. He also made some bizarre flicking actions with his fingers close to his eyes" (Goh & Xie, 2019, p.17). These observable traits were indicative of autism spectrum disorder (ASD), and the condition should be more accurately described as syndromic autism. The reason is that autism or ASD was never BK's primary disorder. BK was only able to engage very briefly with others and after that he returned quickly to his sedentary state. He reinforced and maintained his rejection of eye contact by vibrating his hands in front of his eyes and/or by screaming. On the whole, BK liked all kinds of physical activities and needed constant support of adults (i.e., his teachers and parents) during his days in the kindergarten.

When BK's family was relocated to France due to his father's job posting, it was during that time in Paris that the family discovered BK's gift in music. After hearing a friend play the piano, BK was able to recall the melody and replayed the tune immediately on the piano. However, it was a single occurrence and BK was not subsequently exposed to music or a piano while in Paris and the incident was forgotten. When the family relocated to Frankfurt, the parents hired a piano teacher for BK. It started out well and BK was making progress. "As time progressed, the teacher attempted to introduce new piano books for advanced lessons. BK resisted and became increasingly frustrated leading to a breakdown in the relationship with the piano teacher. BK then abandoned lessons and has not touched a piano since that time" (Camulli, Goh, & Chia, 2018, p.113-114).

The family returned to Singapore in 2002 after BK's father finished his overseas stint. BK was able to join a center that supports youths with autism. Upon reaching 18 years of age, however, he had to leave the center in search of support for adults. The parents reported that he has shown considerable regression since that time.

BK's Family History

When BK was diagnosed with infantile spasms at the age of 10 months, doctors prescribed Prednisolone and Mogadon daily. As a result, the seizures subsided. Plans to tail off the Prednisolone after a few weeks and follow up with another Electroencephalogram (EEG), were not achieved due to the family's decision to relocate to Dubai where the father was given a job posting. This move was the beginning of a 15-year global journey that the family would embark on to accompany the father's continuous redeployment as a station manager for a national airline company in different cities in Europe, Middle East and Asia, such as Dubai, Copenhagen, San Francisco, Paris, Seoul, Frankfurt, and Singapore.

With frequent re-locational changes for BK's family, there were gaps and disturbances in BK's therapeutic support schedule. Moreover, besides the language barrier that BK had to cope with and adapt to in different countries, there were also different treatment approaches to support BK and it was overwhelming for him. Some locations had more services available to provide to BK and the family while others only provided support in their national language or used methods incompatible with BK. Hence, at times, BK made progress, while at other times, he regressed.

In 2002, BK's family returned to Singapore. BK, aged 16 by that time, was able to join a local centre supporting youth with autism. However, when he turned 18 years old, he could no longer be supported by the centre. His parents reported that he had shown a considerable regression since that time. A family friend recommended them to have a new psycho-educational assessment done to know BK's current status and then decide how to support him and consider what options were available to help him to maximize his potential.

According to Goh and Xie (2019), "[B]y the time when BK turned 24 years 3 months, his father had retired from work due to a rare medical condition known as syringomyelia in which a fluid-filled cyst (known as syrinx) forms within the spinal cord" (p.17). "As the syrinx expands and lengthens over time, it compresses and damages part of the spinal cord from its center outward" (Krause, 2019, para.2). It may result in loss of feeling, paralysis, weakness, and stiffness in the back, shoulders, and extremities.

Camulli, Goh and Chia (2018) reported that "BK began to paint in August 2014 when he participated in a church event to paint a mural on the side of the church. Since that time, he has expressed keen interest in painting. Upon a recommendation from a friend, the parents took BK to an art class where he has been going to once a week since that time" (p.114). It soon became evident that BK had a talent for painting and he has since worked to produce many works that give evidence to his eye for detail, colour, texture, and stroke application (Camulli, Goh, & Chia, 2018), as seen in Figures 1 to 6.

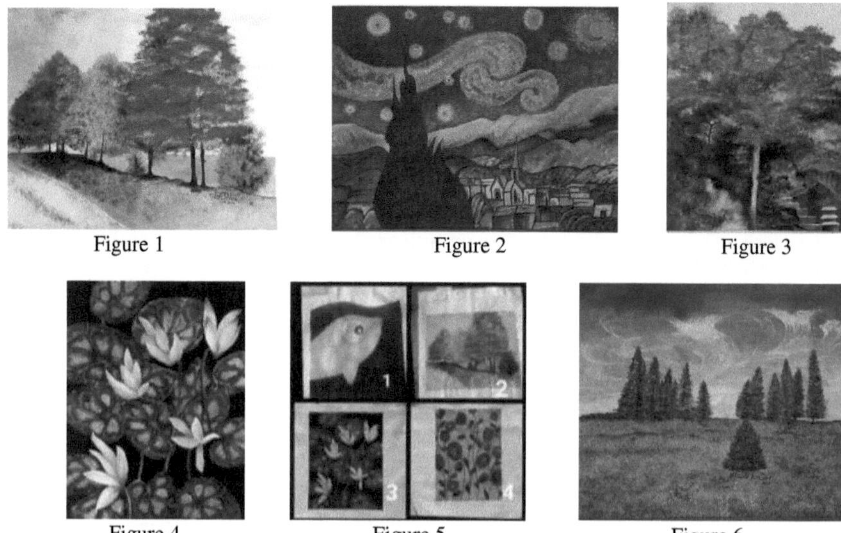

Figure 1   Figure 2   Figure 3

Figure 4   Figure 5   Figure 6

BK's Medical History

According to BK's medical records, he was born at 40 weeks' gestation via forceps delivery in 1986. His weight at the time of birth was 2900g and upon delivery, he underwent phototherapy to treat his severe jaundice.

When BK was about four months old, he had several bouts of fits, especially with a startle response on waking up. Later, it was followed by an increasing number of fits, having more than 5 times per day. "The fits were described as 'salaaming' attacks occurring when he was awake as well as when he was asleep" (Goh & Xie, 2019, p.16). As a result, BK was admitted to a public hospital when he was 10 months old to be treated for infantile spasms (see Shields, 2006, for more detail) by a prominent professor of paediatrics in September 1987. BK was prescribed Prednisolone (20mg) and Mogadon (a quarter of a tablet). As fits began to subside, Prednisolone also started to tail off over a period of several weeks, and BK's parents did not report any further occurrences of his fits. Later, as reported by Goh and Xie (2019), BK underwent an electroencephalogram (EEG) in July 1989. Hypsarrhythmia could be seen on the EEG. "Hypsarrhythmia is a very high-voltage, disorganized pattern of EEG abnormality" (Shields, 2006, p.64). A computed tomography (CT) scan (formerly known as a computerized axial tomography scan or CAT scan) was done at the public hospital and the results revealed periventricular calcifications in his brain, especially in the left occipito-parietal region.

According to Camulli, Goh and Chia (2018) and Goh and Xie (2019), BK's previous medical assessment reports (dated in 1987, 1991 and 2011) from a public hospital in Singapore and another report from a hospital in Denmark diagnosed him with infantile spasms (a frequent and significant cause of morbidity) with hypsarrhythmia and TSC with autistic features (see Chapter Three for more detail).

In February 1990, another EEG was administered and the results showed a spike focus on the right post-temporal occipital lobe reaching the biparietal spreading. It was considered significant for epilepsy and for focal pathology. The EEG pattern was unchanged from the one taken earlier in 1989.

Furthermore, three spots of achromia, which is loss or absence of normal pigmentation (as of the skin), were found on BK's chest and near left axilla (armpit), but there were no shagreen patches (thick, leathery, dimpled lesions) or adenoma sebaceum (red papules that appear on and around the nose, lips, cheeks and chin). In addition, the medical report stated that BK's heart and lungs were clear and his abdomen was noted to be soft. There were no focal neurological signs noted, but BK was found to be developmentally delayed.

From the assessment results (dated 1987, 1991, and 2011), BK was diagnosed with infantile spasms with hypsarrhythmia (see Shields, 2006, for detail) and TSC with autistic features (score in the mildly-moderately autistic area on the Childhood Autism Rating Scale) and extremely low mental capacity (with Performance IQ of 47 at < 0.1 percentile rank with 95% confidence interval between 43 and 57 based on Wechsler Adult Intelligence Scales 3rd Edition/WAIS-III administration). As reported by Camulli, Goh and Chia (2018), "[B]eing non-verbal, BK was unable to complete the WAIS-III assessment and no Verbal IQ and Full-Scale IQ could be computed. In addition, his standard scores based on the administration of Vineland Adaptive Behavior Scales-2nd Edition (VABS-II) showed that his low adaptive behaviour composite score was 26±7 with < 1 percentile rank. The various VABS-II subdomains also showed low standard scores and adaptive levels: Communication = 21±7, Daily Living Skills = 46±8, Socialization = 23±7, and Motor Skills (estimated) = 47±0, all at < 1 percentile rank and low adaptive level. BK was also diagnosed with allergic rhinitis and a lesion in the abdomen ventral to the aorta and inferior vena cava. He was on medication for his epilepsy at that time" (p.112).

According to Camulli, Goh and Chia (2018), BK was reported to undergo an MRI scanning on 20th November 1991 at a public hospital in Copenhagen, Denmark. The MRI uses magnetic fields and radio waves to produce images of thin slices of tissue (tomographic images). During the scanning, the magnitude and rate of energy release that occurs as the protons resume the alignment (T1 relaxation) and as they wobble ("precess") during the process (T2 relaxation) are recorded as spatially localized signal intensities by a coil (antenna) built within the MRI device. Computer algorithms analyse these signals and produce detailed anatomic images. The technique used with BK involved the following:

(i)   T1 weighted sagittal images;
(ii)   T2 weighted axial images;
(iii)   pre- and post-contract T1 weighted axial images; and
(iv)   pre- and post-contrast T1 weighted coronal images (see Figures 7a, 7b and 7c)" (Camulli, Goh, & Chia, 2018, p.112).

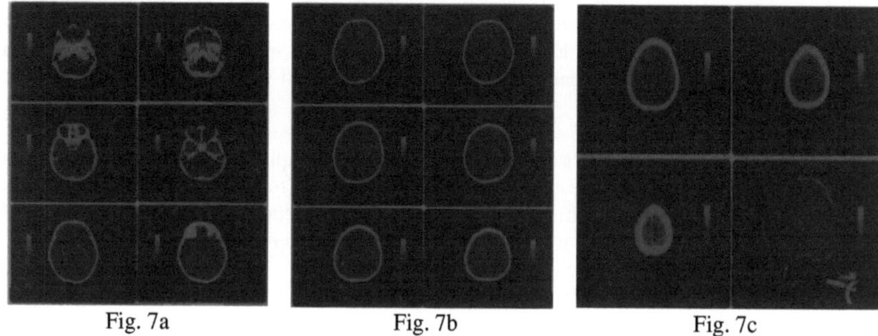

Fig. 7a   Fig. 7b   Fig. 7c

Figure 7. Detection of Intracranial Calcifications by MRI

Camulli, Goh and Chia (2018) reported that "[F]indings from the MRI report indicated that multiple tiny nodules could be found in the subependymal regions of the lateral ventricles bilaterally. None of these nodules had demonstrated enhancement. Focal areas of T2 prolongation were seen in the subcortical white matter and cortex bilaterally. These lesions also failed to show any enhancement following gadolinium contrast. Small (less than 1 cm) cystic structure, which follows CSF[1] signal intensity, was seen posterior to the right lateral ventricle near the splenium. No other definite focal lesions were identified" (p112-113).

In a study conducted by Oot et al. (1986), it was reported that while the MRI images raised the possibility of calcification they were less definitive than the Computed Tomography (CT) findings. In fact, in another earlier study done by Holland et al. (1985), it was reported that calcification was falsely suspected to be present in 45% of non-calcified intracranial abnormalities by MRI. Hence, it is important to err on the side of caution in BK's case especially when one is uncertain of the neuroradiological results.

---

[1] CSF, or cerebrospinal fluid, is a clear, transcellular fluid suitable as an internal signal-intensity reference for gadolinium contrast medium to improve visibility of internal structures for the presence of tumors, subependymal nodules, cortical dysplasias, or subependymal giant cell astrocytomas (SEGAs) during magnetic resonance imaging. For more information, refer to DiMario et al. (2015).

CHAPTER TWO
LITERATURE REVIEW

Introduction

"In the face of a rare disease that results in significant cognitive and social impairment, one could say that to produce remarkable works of art requires 'talent against all odds'. Yet such talent exists and examples have been discovered and verified and the unique elements to each continue to astound both researchers and lay people alike" (Camulli, Goh, & Chia, 2018, p.110). In this monograph, the authors present the research and findings of a young Chinese man with the initials BK, who, despite having Tuberous Sclerosis Complex (TSC) with significant intellectual and developmental impairments, co-existing with syndromic autism, paints extraordinary images of remarkable quality, suggesting he also has Savant Syndrome.

Tuberous Sclerosis Complex

Tuberous Sclerosis Complex (TSC), according to Northrup, Koenig, Pearson and Au (1999), involves abnormalities of the skin (hypomelanotic macules, confetti skin lesions, facial angiofibromas, shagreen patches, fibrous cephalic plaques, ungual fibromas); brain (subependymal nodules, cortical dysplasias, and subependymal giant cell astrocytomas, seizures, intellectual disability and/or developmental delay, psychiatric illness); kidney (angiomyolipomas, cysts, renal cell carcinomas); heart (rhabdomyomas, arrhythmias); and lungs (lymphangioleiomyomatosis, multifocal micronodular pneumonocyte hyperplasia). Central nervous system tumours are the leading cause of morbidity and mortality; renal disease is the second leading cause of early death" (para.1).

The Online Mendelian Inheritance in Man[2] (or OMIM for short; Amberger et al., 2019) has classified TSC as one of the rare diseases in the world with a prevalence affecting approximately 1 in 6000 births. It occurs in all races and ethnic groups and in both males and females. TSC is an autosomal dominant disorder that can be inherited from one parent with TSC or can result from a spontaneous genetic mutation. It is caused by mutations of at least two different genes, the TSC1 gene or the TSC2 gene (Crino, Nathanson, & Henske, 2006), which will be briefly elaborated later. Children have a 50 percent chance of inheriting TSC if one of their parents has this condition, however only one-third of TSC cases are known to be inherited. The other two-thirds result from spontaneous and unpredictable mutations occurring during conception or very early development of the human embryo.

As a result, there are two different types of TSC depending on its genetic causation: TSC1 or TSC2. The OMIM provides two different identification codes: for the Tuberous Sclerosis Complex Type 1 (TSC-1 with a hyphen to distinguish it from its TSC1 gene), its OMIM code is #191100, while for the Tuberous Sclerosis Complex Type 2 (TSC-2 with a hyphen to distinguish it from its TSC2 gene), its OMIM code is #613254. With the addition of the term *complex* – first introduced by the pathologist Moolten (1942) – it gives the emphasis on the multisystemic involvement and variable expression of the disease, and according to the US National Library of Medicine, (2019) the tuberous sclerosis complex (TSC) "affects an estimated of one person in

---

[2] *Online Mendelian Inheritance in Man* (OMIM®) is the continuation of Dr. Victor A. McKusick's *Mendelian Inheritance in Man*, and there were 12 editions in all with the last one published in 1998. It contains an updated catalog of human genes and genetic disorders and traits. Its main focus is on the molecular relationship between genetic variation and phenotypic expression. Currently, OMIM is bio-curated at the McKusick-Nathans Institute of Genetic Medicine, The Johns Hopkins University School of Medicine. For more information, refer to Amberger et al. (2019).

6000" (para.5). The signs and symptoms of the TSC, which "may affect any human organ with well-circumscribed, benign, non-invasive lesions known as hamartias and hamartomas" (Gomez, 1987) vary from person to person. The disease can result in developmental problems and/or even can cause significant health problems to an individual with TSC, especially when it affects kidney, heart and brain.

TSC is a genetic disorder with autosomal dominant inheritance that can affect the brain, heart, skin, kidneys, lungs, and retina (Roach & Sparagana, 2004). It is characterized by the growth of numerous non-cancerous (benign) tumours in different parts of the body caused by mutations in the TSC-1 and/or TSC-2 genes (Huang & Manning, 2008; Knowles, et al, 2003; Sampson, 2003). These two genes play an important role in providing genetic instructions for the making of two essential proteins – hamartin (by TSC1-1) and tuberin (by TSC-2). Within the cells, the two proteins work collaboratively together in modulating cell growth and size. Both hamartin and tuberin serve as tumour suppressors so as to prevent cells from growing and dividing too fast or in an uncontrolled way that results in tumorous growth. In other words, with the loss of these two proteins due to TSC-1 and TSC-2 mutation, cells will grow and divide uncontrollably resulting in a tumour. The loss of hamartin or tuberin in different types of cells causes tumours in many different tissues or organs.

According to the US National Library of Medicine (2019) individuals with TSC "are born with one mutated copy of the TSC-1 (OMIM #191100) or TSC-2 (OMIM #613254) gene in each cell. This mutation prevents the cell from making functional hamartin or tuberin from the altered copy of the gene" (para.7). In about 33% of the TSC cases, an individual can inherit an altered TSC-1 or TSC-2 gene from his/her parent who has the disease. The remaining 67% of the TSC cases happen in individuals with no history of TSC in their families.

Manifestations of TSC

The TSC-1 mutations are more common in familial cases of TSC while the TSC-2 mutations occur more sporadically. In fact, the TSC-2 mutation causes most cases of lymphangioleiomyomatosis (LAM for short) – a devastating lung disease (characterized by the abnormal overgrowth of smooth muscle-like tissue in the lungs) that occurs almost exclusively in women, causing coughing, shortness of breath, chest pain, and lung collapse (Carsillo, Astrinidis, & Henske, 2000; Chorianopoulos & Stratakos, 2008; Goncharova & Krymskaya, 2008).

Generally, all individuals with TSC have skin abnormalities, "including patches of unusually light-colored skin, areas of raised and thickened skin, and growths under the nails" (US National Library of Medicine, 2019). Tumours that appear on the face are known as facial angiofibromas and these are common at the start of the condition in childhood.

Kidney tumours are common in individuals with TSC. These tumours can affect kidney functions, resulting in serious life-threatening problems, such as end-stage renal failure (Clarke et al., 1999) acute kidney failure (Siroky, Yin, & Bissler, 2010) renal angiomyolipomas (Wilson et al., 2005) pyelonephritis and polycystic kidney disease (Mohkam et al., 2014). Moreover, tumours can develop in the heart (Tuberous Sclerosis Association, 2017a) resulting in cardiac rhabdomyomas (Wilson et al., 2005) as well as tumours developing in the liver, lungs, teeth and mouth, and the light-sensitive tissue at the back of the eye (the retina) (Tuberous Sclerosis Association, 2017b).

The brain is also another vital organ that is often affected by TSC and the resulting benign (non-cancerous) tumours in the brain can cause serious or life-threatening complications. There are several cerebral abnormalities associated with TSC: cortical tubers, subependymal nodules

(SEN), subependymal giant cell tumours (SGCT), and white matter abnormalities such as radial bands and wedge-shaped lesions (Bozzao, Manenti, & Curatolo, 2003; DiMario, 2004; Griffiths, Bolton, & Verity, 1998). In many cases, TSC has caused "seizures, behavioral problems such as hyperactivity and aggression, and intellectual disability or learning problems" (US National Library of Medicine, 2019). There are also reported cases (e.g., Deweerdt, 2014; Lewis et al., 2013; Guo, Tu, & Shi, 2012) of children with TSC manifesting the autistic features, such as impairment in communication and social interaction.

As TSC causes typically benign tubers (hamartia) or tumours (hamartomas) to grow on vital organs, this can lead to a wide range of physical and neuropsychiatric disorders. Epilepsy is present in 70%-90% of individuals with TSC and often develops within the first year of life. Developmental and behavioural disorders including autism spectrum conditions (ASC) or autism spectrum disorders (ASD), are also frequently diagnosed in TSC (Prather & de Vries, 2004). According to research studies, ASC affects between 17% and 63% of individuals with TSC, a prevalence dramatically higher than that of the general population (Ridler, Suckling, Higgins, de Vries, Stephenson, Bolton, & Bullmore, (2007). Mental retardation and early onset of epilepsy in TSC, in particular infantile spasms, are associated with the development of ASC/ASD in such individuals. In addition, there is evidence of an association between temporal lobe epileptiform foci with ASC/ASD in TSC. Self-injurious behaviour and other behaviours such as ADHD, aggression, behavioural outbursts and obsessive compulsive disorder (OCD) can also occur in some patients with TSC (Staley, Montenegro, Major, Muzykewicz, Halpern, Kopp, Newberry, & Thiele, 2008).

An estimated 17 to 61 percent of individuals with TSC manifest symptoms of autism (Asano et al., 2000). Other neurological symptoms, as already mentioned above, commonly seen in such individuals also include epilepsy, intellectual disability, challenging behaviours and developmental impairment (Crino, Nathanson, & Henske, 2006; Lewis et al., 2013). Several studies have shown that cortical tubers, which are developmental abnormalities of the cerebral cortex (Umeoka et al., 2008) found in individuals with TSC, are related to epilepsy and are foci for seizures. In fact, cortical tubers have been reported in 82% to 100% of people with TSC (Ridler et al., 2004).

In a study done by Gallagher et al. (2010) three types of cortical tubers, which widely vary in size, appearance and location, were identified based on the MRI signal intensity of the subcortical white matter component in individuals with TSC (see Table 1 below).

Table 1. Three Cortical Tuber Types as identified by MRI

Tubers Type	Description
Cortical Tuber Type #A	These cortical tubers are isointense on volumetric T1 images and subtly hyperintense on T2 weighted and fluid-attenuated inversion recovery.
Cortical Tuber Type #B	These cortical tubers are hypointense on volumetric T1 images and homogeneously hyperintense on T2 weighted and fluid-attenuated inversion recovery (FLAIR).
Cortical Tuber Type #C	These cortical tubers are hypointense on volumetric T1 images, hyperintense on T2 weighted, and heterogeneous on FLAIR characterized by a hypointense central region surrounded by a hyperintense rim.

Source: Gallagher et al. (2010).

The relationship between cortical tuber features and clinical phenotype remains unclear. Based on the dominant cortical tuber types present, Gallagher et al. (2010) identified three distinct groups of people with each of the three cortical tuber types. Those with dominant Cortical Tuber Type #A manifest a milder phenotype. Those with dominant Cortical Type #C tuber show more MRI abnormalities (e.g., subependymal giant cell tumours) with a higher chance of having autism spectrum disorder, a history of infantile spasms, and a higher frequency of epileptic seizures, compared to those who have a dominant Cortical Tuber Type #B, and especially to those with dominant Cortical Tuber Type #A. However, it is not within the scope of this monograph to delve on this issue.

Autism Spectrum Disorders

The original concept of autism was developed by Bleuler (1911, 1978) and the disorder was then a symptom of schizophrenia, which was coined by Bleuler himself. According to Bleuler (1911), autism is a symptom related to the psychopathology of (i) dementia praecox[3] (Kraepelin, 1887a, 1887b), which was believed to be primarily a disease of the brain – or (ii) the group of schizophrenias[4], i.e., a cerebral disease with primary symptoms in the disturbances of four 'a's: *a*ssociations, *a*ffect, *a*mbivalence and *a*utistic isolation.

The first version of the Diagnostic and Statistical Manual (DSM) of mental disorders, published by the American Psychological Association (APA), appeared in 1952, building upon the statistical data and classification system developed by the U.S. Army in post-World War II America as well as the sixth edition of International Classification of Diseases (ICD) published by the World Health Organization. Autism first appeared in the DSM in 1980 under the label Infantile Autism (DSM History, 2018).

The diagnostic criteria used for Autism Spectrum Disorder (ASD) has changed over the past decades with improved understanding of this complex developmental disability. The DSM has responded to the evolving understanding of ASD by issuing updated definitions in each new edition to reflect the collective knowledge. Only in its most recent edition, DSM-V, was autism renamed Autism Spectrum Disorder not only to more accurately reflect the wide range [spectrum] of symptoms, manifestations, skills, and levels of disability but also to facilitate diagnosis by focusing on the shared principal characteristics of the different phenotypes of ASD rather than their differences. Table 2 shows some changes in the DSM diagnostic criteria over a period of time from 1980 to 2013 with the publication of the fifth edition DSM.

Table 2. Changes in the DSM Diagnostic Criteria for ASD: 1980-2013

DSM-III (1980)	DSM-III-R (1987)	DSM-IV (1994) DSM-IV-TR (2000)	DSM-5 (2013)
Infantile Autism	**Autistic Disorder**	**Autistic Disorder**	**Autism Spectrum Disorder (ASD)**
Onset before 30 months	Onset before 36 months	Delays or abnormal functioning in one area (social interaction,	Symptoms in early developmental period (may not manifest until

---

[3] Kraepelin (1887a, 1887b) distinguished dementia praecox from other forms of dementia (such as Alzheimer's disease) which typically occur late in life.

[4] Bleuler (1911) emphasized the notion of a fundamental disorder of thought and feeling in his concept of schizophrenia.

		language or play) before 36 months	social demands exceed limited capacities)
Gross deficits in language development	Qualitative impairment in both verbal and nonverbal communication	Qualitative impairment in communication	Persistent deficits in social communication and social interaction
Pervasive lack of responsiveness to others	Qualitative impairment in reciprocal social interaction	Qualitative impairment in social interaction	Deficits in social-emotional reciprocity and social relationships

Formerly (DSM-IV and/or DSM-IV-TR[5]), the types of autism that now fall under the collective umbrella of ASD, were listed as separate but related disorders under the broad diagnosis of Pervasive Development Disorders. These include Autistic Disorder, Asperger's Disorder, and Pervasive Development Disorder–Not Otherwise Specified (PDD-NOS). These are now subsumed within ASD, or, in some cases of higher functioning individuals who do not exhibit all of the requisite criteria for the diagnosis of ASD, reclassified under Social Communication Disorder (SCD) (Lai, Lombardo, Chakrabarti, & Baron-Cohen, 2013). Still absent, however, is the mention of autistic savant or savant syndrome from the DSM-5. This will be addressed further on in this monograph.

Studies by Gibbs, Aldridge, Chandler, Witzlsperger, and Smith (2012) and Huerta, Bishop, Duncan, Hus, and Lord (2012) have both shown that DSM-5 provides better specificity to reduce false-positive diagnoses, but at the expense of potentially reducing sensitivity, especially for older children, adolescents, and adults, individuals without intellectual disability, and individuals who previously met criteria for diagnoses of DSM-IV Asperger's Disorder or PDD-NOS.

Although some previously distinct diagnoses have been eliminated or absorbed by the ASD designation, the DSM-5 does offer distinctions within the ASD umbrella to reflect level of severity of symptoms. The three severity levels are based on the level of support needed, due to challenges with social communication and restricted interests and repetitive behaviours. Table 3 presents the descriptors used as qualitative criteria for determining the diagnostic level of ASD of an individual. The inclusion of levels of severity and the relative vagueness that prevails within each description further reflects the range (i.e., spectrum) of manifest challenges observed and experienced in the autistic population. These changes highlight the varied nature of the two primary behaviour domains of ASD, and improve the organization of symptom descriptions with the aim of reducing or eliminating misdiagnoses or conflicting diagnoses among clinicians (Lai et al., 2013). However, Camulli and Goh (2018) argued, "But are they enough?" (p.186).

Table 3. Severity Levels in DSM-5 for ASD Diagnosis and Coding

Severity Level for ASD	Social Communication	Restricted Interests & Repetitive Behaviours (RRBs)
Level 3	Severe deficits in verbal and nonverbal social communication skills cause severe impairments in functioning; very limited initiation of social interaction and	Preoccupations, fixated rituals and/or repetitive behaviours markedly interfere with functioning in all spheres. Marked distress when rituals or routines are

---

[5] TR stands for Text Revision.

'Requiring very substantial support'	minimal response to social overtures from others.	interrupted; very difficult to redirect from fixated interest or returns to it quickly.
Level 2 'Requiring substantial support'	Marked deficits in verbal and nonverbal social communication skills; social impairments apparent even with supports in place; limited initiation of social interactions and reduced or abnormal response to social overtures from others	RRBs and/or preoccupations or fixated interests appear frequently enough to be obvious to the casual observer and interfere with functioning in a variety of contexts. Distress or frustration is apparent when RRBs are interrupted; difficult to redirect from fixated interest.
Level 1 'Requiring support'	Without supports in place, deficits in social communication cause noticeable impairments. Has difficulty initiating social interactions and demonstrates clear examples of atypical or unsuccessful responses to social overtures of others. May appear to have decreased interest in social interactions.	Rituals and repetitive behaviours (RRBs) cause significant interference with functioning in one or more contexts. Resists attempts by others to interrupt RRBs or to be redirected from fixated interest.

The changes to the DSM-5 serve clinicians in facilitating a diagnosis, in determining qualification for services, and in guaranteeing individuals with required levels of support, but how does this unitary label account for and address the specific and heterogeneous needs of each child with autism and the families, teachers, and therapists who support them? Lai et al (2013) argue that given the known massive heterogeneity within the overarching label of ASD, not just in terms of severity and combination of behavioural symptoms but also in cognition and biological mechanisms, this approach is not useful for research in general nor for identifying and addressing the partially distinct aetiologies [and comorbidities].

Lai and his team (2013) suggest that the term 'spectrum' holds several meanings and that the differences, though subtle, are not trivial. The first refers to the dimensional nature of the cardinal features of autism within the clinical population (i.e., differences in the severity and presentation of symptoms among those with a diagnosis of ASD. The second refers to the continuity between the general population and the clinical population. This perspective of the spectrum necessitates the inclusion of autistic conditions or traits or even associated features that manifest through the whole population. The third meaning refers to subgroups, in contrast to the DSM-V that intentionally tried to move away from focusing on the differences by emphasizing the essential shared features of the autism spectrum. His team offers an expanded, though not exhaustive, list of 'specifiers' to further differentiate individuals within the ASD population. Table 4 outlines examples from the list of specifiers Lai and his team (2013) propose to assist in the identification of subgroups.

Table 4. Sample List of Specifiers toward the Identification of ASD Subgroups

Category	Specifier	Example
Developmental patterns	Pattern of atypical development	1.Age and pattern of onset/regression 2.Trajectory of development 3.Language Onset 4.Hyperlexia
Sex/gender	Biological sex	Male/female
	Sex/gender-adjusted autistic features	Statistical characterization of autistic trait (e.g., percentile) relative to sex/gender-specific norms
Clinical phenotype	Co-occurring condition	1.Epilepsy 2.Macrocephaly 3.Immune disorders 4.Attention deficit/hyperactivity disorder 5. Dyslexia 6. Sleep disruption
	Taxonomic formulation	1.Asperger Syndrome 2.Aloof/passive/active but odd/loners group
Cognitive profile	Intelligence	1.IQ profile 2.Savant memory 3.Savant spatial skills
	Social cognition	1.Emotion perception and understanding 2.Face recognition 3.Emotional contagion
	Executive function	1.Cognitive flexibility 2.Planning 3.Inhibitory control
Genetic	Syndromic autism	1.Fragile X syndrome 2.Rett syndrome 3.Tuberous sclerosis complex

It could be argued that with most of the examples given, a new wave of 'spectrum' exists. For example, the age of language onset can range from very early to late onset to not at all (i.e., the individual has remained non-verbal), or the IQ profile can be spread from moderate mental retardation to above-average intelligence, or the presence of tumours in Tuberous Sclerosis Complex can be minimal or multiple. It stands to reason why the DSM-5 opted to focus on broad similarities of cardinal behavioural domains for the myriad of other co-existing factors complicate, if not distract, the diagnostic process. Lai et al (2013) disagree, concerned that the umbrella term ASD risks whitewashing the evident heterogeneity, simply moving us from the level of subgroups ("apples and oranges") to the prototypical level ("fruit").

A Possible Link between Tuberous Sclerosis Complex and Autism?

In a first long-term assessment of children with TSC, Jeste et al. (2014) identified early markers of autism risk in this group of individuals. It was found that children with TSC and ASD showed a gradual drop in their non-verbal intelligence between one and three years of age, while those with only TSC and without ASD did not manifest this decline (Jeste et al, 2014). As mentioned earlier above, individuals with the dominant Cortical Tuber Type #C have a higher possibility of being diagnosed with secondary or syndromic autism and the authors of this monograph inferred that it could be the case.

According to Deweerdt (2014), who cited from several other studies (i.e., Jeste et al, 2013; Landa et al., 2012; Nie, Di Nardo & Han, 2010), the findings show that children with TSC manifest developmental delays by 6 months of age and they often display difficulties with fine motor and visual skills. These infants are unable to track objects with their eyes and often disengage their attention from one object to look at another. In other words, children with TSC have structural problems in their visual system (Nie, Di Nardo, & Han, 2010). Infants diagnosed with TSC also display differences in face processing similar to those seen in ASD (Jeste et al., 2013). As a result, Jeste et al. (2014) found such early symptoms evolving into more global developmental difficulties by the time these infants were 9-12 months old. With faulty visual system, social interaction will be impaired as the infants grow and develop. One explanation is that the sensory processing abnormalities are feeding into the future social abnormalities (Jeste et al., 2014).

By the age of 3 years old, more than 50% of the participating children in the study done by Jeste et al. (2014) met the diagnostic criteria for ASD. There were also those children with TSC who did not meet the ASD criteria and the study found that this group of children also manifested social deficits. Examining the scores obtained from the assessment, Jeste et al. (2014) found that at 12 months of age, children diagnosed with TSC and ASD scored lower IQ than those with TSC alone. There was also a significant decline in non-verbal IQ over the period between one and three years.

Interestingly, the findings from Jeste's et al. (2014) study have shown that TSC may provide a model specifically of ASD that occurs along with intellectual disability (ID). The model offers a new perspective in better understanding of the relationship between ASD and ID via TSC.

Another Link between Autism and Savant Syndrome?

In the case study of BK, Camulli and Goh (2018) and Camulli, Goh and Chia (2018) reported BK with TSC and syndromic autism to be an autistic savant artist despite his moderate intellectual and developmental disability. According to Chia (2012) autism or autism spectrum disorder (ASD) is defined as "a neuro-developmental syndrome of constitutional origin (genetic) and whose cause could also be epigenetic, and its onset is usually around first three years of birth, with empathizing or mentalizing deficits that result in a triad of impairments in communication, social interaction, and imagination, with manifestation of repetitive stereotyped behaviours, but may, on the other hand, display (especially by autistic savants) or hide (especially by autistic crypto-savants) a strong systemizing drive that accounts for a distinct triad of strengths in good attention to detail, deep narrow interests, and islets of ability" (p.239). In other words, any individual diagnosed with ASD (be it primary, secondary or syndromic autism) can be a savant but that depends on his/her level of systemizing ability.

Talents in autism come in many forms, but a common characteristic is that the individual becomes an expert in recognizing repeating patterns in stimuli or attaining "an excellent understanding of a whole system, given the opportunity to observe and control all the variables in that system" (Baron-Cohen et al., 2009). This systemizing is defined as the drive to analyse or construct systems. These might be any kind of system. What defines a system is that it follows rules, and when we systemize, we are trying to identify the rules that govern the system, in order to predict how that system will behave (Baron-Cohen 2006). Here are some examples of the major kinds of systems:

- Collectible systems (e.g. distinguishing between types of stones or wood);
- Mechanical systems (e.g. a video recorder or a window lock);
- Numerical systems (e.g. a train timetable or a calendar);
- Abstract systems (e.g. the syntax of a language or musical notation);
- Natural systems (e.g. the weather patterns or tidal wave patterns);
- Social systems (e.g. a management hierarchy or a dance routine with a dance partner); and
- Motoric systems (e.g. throwing a Frisbee or bouncing on a trampoline).

In addition to the abovementioned, there are still many other kinds of systems including sensory systems (e.g., tapping surfaces or letting sand run through one's fingers), spatial systems (e.g., obsession with routes), vocal/auditory/verbal systems (e.g., echoing sounds), and systemizing action sequences (e.g., watching the same video repeatedly).

In other words, autistic savants are individuals with a combination of ASD and savant syndrome who display superior systemizing or hyper-systemizing abilities. However, this systemizing should be taken as "part of the cognitive style of people with autism spectrum conditions (ASC)" (Baron-Cohen et al., 2009). With superior systemizing ability in addition to a special talent possessed by an individual with ASD, autistic savant syndrome (or autistic savantism) comes into existence and it is as real as it is rare, but the extraordinary condition with serious mental or intellectual and developmental disabilities possesses some kind of miraculous genius that "stands in marked, incongruous contrast to overall handicap" (Treffert, 2010, p.1).

Savant Syndrome

The phenomenology of Savant Syndrome confirms that it is a rare, enigmatic condition. According to Treffert (2010), "[S]avant [S]yndrome is a rare, but extraordinary, condition in which persons with serious mental disabilities, including autistic disorder, have some 'island of genius' that stands in marked, incongruous contrast to overall handicap" (p.1). The prevalence in the autistic population is approximately 10% and markedly fewer (1%) among non-autistics but who have developmental disabilities (Treffert, 2014). In other words, approximately 50% of cases with Savant Syndrome have autism as the underlying developmental disability and 50% are associated with other disabilities. Unlike TSC, which is represented impartially between genders, males with Savant Syndrome outnumber their female counterparts by as many as six to one (Treffert, 2010).

Savant Syndrome is hallmarked by the paradoxical special skills amidst discernible disability or handicap. In his research, Treffert (2009) identified that remarkable skills are found in only a relatively narrow discrete range of five general categories: (1) Music, usually performance based and most often the piano; (2) Art, usually drawing, painting or sculpting; (3) Mathematics; including lightning calculating or the ability to compute prime numbers, for example, in the absence of other simple arithmetic abilities; (4) Calendar calculating, which is an obscure skill in non-savants and; (5) Mechanical or spatial skills, including the capacity to measure distances precisely without benefit of instruments, the ability to construct complex models or structures with painstaking accuracy or the mastery of map making and direction finding.

Some other skills have also been reported, although less often, such as knowing the time without having to look at a clock, an uncanny ability to know and understand how animals feel, unusual sensory discrimination in smell, touch, or vision including synaesthesia, prodigious language (polyglot) ability, untaught mechanical or computer literacy skills, an unexplainable capability to commit maps to memory, outstanding knowledge in specific fields such as neurophysiology, statistics or navigation, and so on (Chia, 2008). Typically, a single special skill exists, however, in some instances several skills exist simultaneously. Whatever the particular savant skill, it is always linked to phenomenal, sometimes eidetic memory (Treffert, 2006).

"The prevalence of savant syndrome is approximately 10% in the autistic population and less than 1% in the non-autistic population, making the combination rare" (Camulli, Goh, & Chia, 2018). In fact, '[S]avantism is found more commonly in ASC than in any other neurological group (Howlin, Goode, & Hutton, 2009) and the majority of those with savantism have an ASC (Hermelin, 2002)" (Baron-Cohen et al., 2009). Camulli and Goh (2018) have argued that if an individual with TSC manifests autistic traits and at the same time is a savant, the condition is not savant syndrome or ASD. It should be recognized as a combination of both as a syndromic disorder to TSC. In other words, Camulli and Goh (2018) have coined the term *autistic spectrum syndromic disorder* to describe the comorbid condition of TSC.

Exkorn (2005) classifies autistic savant skills into three categories: (1) Splinter skills, (2) Talented skills, and; (3) Prodigious skills. Splinter skills are most common and savants with these skills display obsessive preoccupations with and memorization of trivia and obscure information such as license plate numbers of vehicles and sports statistics, which they commit to memory. Talented skills are more highly developed and specialized than splinter skills. Savants with talented skills can be very artistic and draw or paint beautiful sceneries, or for some, have a fantastic memory that allows them to work out difficult mathematical calculations mentally. Prodigious skills are the rarest. Prodigious savants have spectacular skills that would be remarkable even if they were to occur in non-handicapped individuals. Fewer than 30 known prodigious savants in the world display such extraordinary skills, which could include for instance, the capability to play an entire concerto on the piano after listening to it only once (Chia, 2008).

In summary, there are several features that distinguish a savant artist from other artists: the underlying disability; innate ability without teaching or training; talent which typically 'explodes' on the scene at a very early age; obsessive preoccupation with the skill; prolific output of product on a continuous basis; and literal, eidetic-like memory with massive capacity in the area of expertise (Treffert, 2010).

Savant Syndrome in Autism Spectrum Disorder?

The latest Diagnostic and Statistical Manual of Mental Disorders-5th Edition (DSM-5) (American Psychological Association, 2013) ushered in significant revisions not seen since the last publication of the DSM-IV almost 20 years earlier in 1994 and later in 2003 with its text revision resulting in the DSM-IV-TR. Largely informed by advancements in neuroscience, clinical and public health need, and identified problems with the classification system and criteria put forth in the DSM-IV, the changes to diagnostic criteria for several complex developmental disorders, including autism, have great clinical impact and reflect the evolutionary nature of pinpointing the specific criteria that hallmark such disorders (Regier, Kuhl, & Kupfer, 2013).

In light of this understanding that definitions, criteria, and new insights of developmental disorders continue to emerge, we propose a re-conceptualizing of autistic savantism as a spectrum syndromic disorder.

As already mentioned earlier, the hallmark of savant syndrome (SS) is the paradoxical special skills amidst discernible disability or handicap (Camulli, Goh, & Chia, 2018), and the condition is considered "a rare, but extraordinary … with serious mental disabilities, including autistic disorder, have some 'island of genius' that stands in marked, incongruous contrast to overall handicap" (Treffert, 2010, p. 1).

An undeniable link to the spectrum disorder of autism (or ASD), approximately 50% of cases with savant syndrome have autism as the underlying developmental disability and 50% are associated with other disabilities (Treffert, 2014). As such, this distinction fundamentally expands the operating definition of autism to include autistic savants. Autistic or not, savants can be further categorized into various types, or a 'spectrum' of savantism.

Although savantism (either as autistic savant or savant syndrome) is not yet included in the DSM-5, it has been observed, researched and diagnosed even before John Langdon Down first coined the term 'idiot savant' in a lecture before the Medical Society of London in 1887 (Treffert, 2009). The first known description of savant syndrome in a scientific paper was in the German psychology journal, Know Thyself or Journal of Empirical Psychology (Gnothi Sauton oder Magazin zur Erfahrungsseelenkunde), in 1783 describing the case of an Englishman Jedediah Buxton who was a 'lightning calculator' (Treffert, 2009). Scores of reports since that time describe individuals who have perplexed researchers by their apparent inability to 'comprehend scarcely anything, either theoretical or practical' and yet demonstrate remarkable skill or talent in one, sometimes more, narrow area of interest (Treffert, 2009).

An Expanded Operating Definition of Autism

According to an expanded operating definition of autism or ASD proposed by Chia (2008a), the term ASD is defined "as a neurodevelopmental syndrome of constitutional origin (i.e., genetic and epigenetic causes), whose onset is usually around first three years of birth, with empathizing or mentalizing deficits that result in a triad of impairments in communication, social interaction, and imagination, but may, on the other hand, display (especially by autistic savants) or hide (especially by autistic crypto-savants) a strong systemizing drive that accounts for a distinct triad of strengths in good attention to detail, deep narrow interests, and islets of ability" (p. 10).

It is the second part of the operating definition, i.e., "may … display (especially by autistic savants) or hide (especially by autistic crypto-savants) a strong systemizing drive that accounts for a distinct triad of strengths in good attention to detail, deep narrow interests, and islets of ability" (Chia, 2008a, p. 10), that provides us some kind of an imbedded condition in which someone with significant mental disabilities can still demonstrate certain abilities far in excess of average (Miller, 1999; Treffert, 2009). Although it seems like there are two extreme ends apart between autistic crypto-savants per se and autistic savants per se, whatever falls in between them constitutes a spectrum of savant abilities including those with splinter skills, talented skills and prodigious skills (Exkorn, 2005). We have decided to term this spectrum disorder of autistic savants as autistic savant spectrum syndromic disorder or ASSSD for short (see Figure 8).

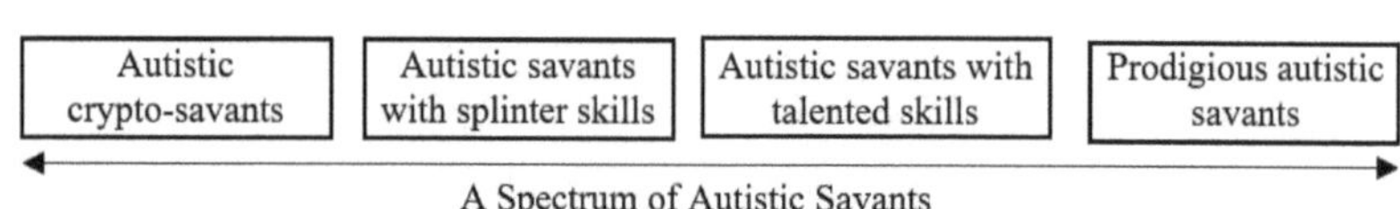

Figure 8. Autistic Savant Spectrum Syndromic Disorder

Autistic Savant Spectrum Syndromic Disorder

When several disabilities/disorders share certain key [autistic] symptoms, they constitute a *syndrome* (Chia & Camulli, 2017, p. 136). In ASSSD, *syndrome* is the third S-word to be added to the term with the first S-word being *savant*. According to Şıklar and Berberoğlu (2014), the term *syndrome* refers "to a group of specific features which appear to be unrelated, but which define a number of disorders when they develop together" (p. 1). Also known as *syndromic disorder* (see Figure 9), it involves a combination of symptoms resulting from a single cause or so commonly occurring together as to constitute a distinct clinical *disorder*. One good example is the generalized attention behavioural syndrome (GABS) (see Figure 10).

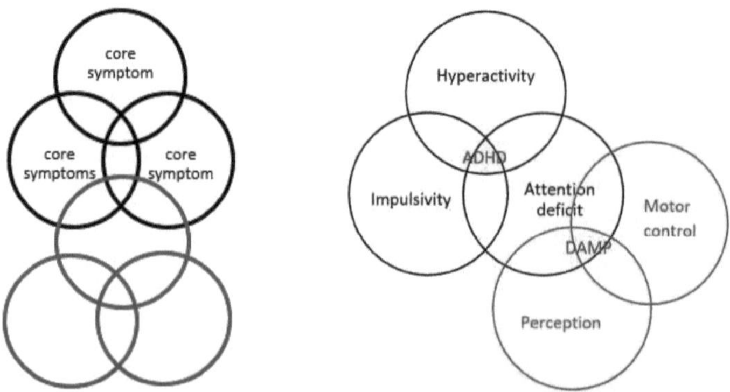

Figure 9. A Model of a Syndromic Disorder

Figure 10. Generalized Attention Behavioural Syndrome

It consists of inattention as the key common symptom shared by two other disorders: (1) Attention Deficit Hyperactivity Disorder (ADHD) with three core symptoms namely, inattention, hyperactivity and impulsivity (see Rydelius, 2000, for detail); and (2) the Deficits in Attention, Motor control and Perception (DAMP)[6] (see Gillberg, 2003; Landgren, Kjellman, & Gillberg, 2000, for detail). Other examples include Angelman Syndrome, Noonan Syndrome and Prader-Willi syndrome.

Within the syndromic disorder of autistic savants, there is spectrum of several distinct categories or classes since they fall within the same continuum. Hence, the second S-word

---

[6] The concept of DAMP was first introduced as a variant of minimal brain dysfunction (MBD) (Rydelius, 2000, p. 266). Up to this day, there is still no official diagnostic code for DAMP. Figure 2 shows a model of a syndromic disorder.

spectrum is added to the ASSSD. On one end of the spectrum is a group of autistic crypto-savants, a term coined by Rimland (1990) to describe those autistic savants "because of their inability to communicate, who have savant skills that are hidden and unknown to all around them" (p.3). Very little has been written about or researched on autistic crypto-savants since the time when Rimland (1990) reported the phenomenon and backed up with three cases that he had encountered.

The next group on the spectrum is the autistic savants with splinter skills, being the most common of all. These autistic savants manifest obsessive preoccupations with and memorization of trivia and obscure information (Siegel, 1996), e.g., license plate numbers of vehicles and names of all the recent and past soccer players in the Manchester United FC, which they commit to memory. However, according to Young (2005), "[T]he term splinter skill is ... used to describe a skill that is extraordinary only in comparison to one's overall functioning. These skills are more common among the autistic population and typically involve memory for facts. Individuals demonstrating only splinter skills do not warrant 'savant' classification" (p. 200).

Treffert (1989, 2000) provides a useful distinction for the savants with regard to their competence level of skill and he uses the two terms "talented savant" and "prodigious savant" to describe the two categories of savantism. In other words, falling within the savant spectrum is a group of autistic savants with talented skills who have a more highly developed and specialized skill. Often, they are found to be very artistic and paint beautiful sceneries or draw detailed images (Camulli, Goh, & Chia, 2018; Selfe, 1977; Wiltshire, 1989). For some of them, they have a fantastic memory that allows them to work out difficult mathematical calculations mentally (Chia, 2008b; Tammet, 2006). The other group that follows after and falls on the other end of the spectrum constitutes the prodigious savants, being the rarest type (see Barlow, 1952; Goldsmith, 1987). They possess spectacular skills that would be remarkable even if they were to occur in non-handicapped individuals. "It is likely, however, that a prodigious savant represents an extreme instance within a continuum of skills rather than a discrete category" (Young, 2005, p. 200). According to the Better Health Channel (February 2007), there are only about 25 such prodigious savants in the world; for instance, the capability of a prodigious savant to play an entire concerto on the piano after listening it only once (Charness, Clifton, & MacDonald, 1988).

Underlying these savant abilities or extraordinary skills is that incredible systemizing ability to analyse and build systems so as to understand and predict the functional behaviour of impersonal events or inanimate or abstract entities (Chia, 2008a, p. 3-4). Myers, Baron-Cohen and Wheelwright (2004) have listed the following six systems: (1) mechanical systems such as machines and tools (see Brink, 1979; Hoffman & Reeves, 1979); (2) natural systems such as biological processes (e.g., respiration) and geographical phenomena (e.g., earthquakes) (see Grandin, 2000; Grandin & Johnson, 2005); (3) abstract systems such as mathematical concepts (e.g., integration, 3x3 matrices) and computer programs (including digital games) (see Brill, 1940; Chia, 2008c); (4) motoric systems such as 3-D drawing, piano finger technique or a lawn tennis shot (see Charness, Clifton, & MacDonald, 1988; Selfe, 1977); (5) organizable systems such as Dewey Classification System used in library catalogue or a stamp collection (see Chia, 2007; Shah & Frith, 1993); and (6) social systems such as a business management or a football team (see Golan & Baron-Cohen, 2006; Lawson, 2001).

CHAPTER THREE
PSYCHO-EDUCATIONAL ASSESSMENT, EVALUATION AND PROFILING

This chapter provides an overview with some details on the psycho-educational assessments that BK had undergone on three different occasions: 1994, 2011 and 2018.

First Set of Psycho-educational Assessment Results

In July, 1994, BK's mother requested for a psychological assessment/evaluation to be done in order to assist her in planning ahead for BK's education when the family returned to Singapore with the father from overseas attachment. Because of his developmental delay, the following several assessments were administered when he was back in Singapore: Leiter International Performance Scale-Revised (LIPS-R; Roid, et al., 1997) the Vineland Adaptive Behavior Scales-Interview Edition (VABS-I; Sparrow, Cicchetti, & Balla, 1984) the *Beery-Buktenica* Developmental Test for Visual-Motor Integration (VMI; Beery, 1997) and the Childhood Autism Rating Scale (CARS; Schopler, Reichier, & Renner, 1988). For the description for each of these assessment tools, interested readers can refer to The Special Educator's Comprehensive Guide to 301 Diagnostic Tests (Pierangelo & Giuliani, 2006).

No assessment report with quantitative data was provided. Only a descriptive write-up reporting on BK's results obtained from the cross-battery assessment (X-BA) was given. The X-BA approach uses multiple test batteries in guiding the diagnostic decision (Flanagan & McGrew, 1997) to gain a more complete understanding of BK's cognitive and behavioural abilities. The results are briefly discussed below:

Leiter International Performance Scale-Revised (LIPS-R)

On the LIPS-R (Roid, et al., 1997) administration, there was little success in engaging BK. According to his psychological assessment report, BK's scores fell the standard score of 50 and that indicated that he was intellectually challenged.

Vineland Adaptive Behavior Scales-Interview Edition (VABS-I)

The VABS-I (Sparrow, Cicchetti, & Balla, 1984) was utilized to assess BK's adaptive functioning. Information regarding his adaptive behaviour was obtained through an interview with both his classroom teacher and his mother. The results covered four domains: (i) communication, (ii) activities of daily living, (iii) socialization, and (iv) motor skills. All the four domains were reported to be in the range between Moderately Low and Low. His adaptive behaviour composite was in the "Low" category. His adaptive functioning level was noted to be in the limited intellectual functioning range.

Beery-Buktenica Developmental Test for Visual-Motor Integration (VMI)

As reported by Camulli, Goh and Chia (2018), BK was able to accurately draw vertical and horizontal lines in the Beery-Buktenica Developmental Test of Visual-Motor Integration (Beery, 1997). However, in 2018, when BK was asked to draw a person as in the Draw-A-Person Intellectual Ability Test (DAP-IQ; Reynolds & Hickman, 2004), which is a systematic and standardized method for evaluating an examinee's process used in a common drawing task to evaluate cognitive abilities, he was unable to do so. He could only produce random scribbles but no schemata of human figure, tree or house were noted in his projective drawings.

Childhood Autism Rating Scale (CARS)

The results obtained from the CARS (Schopler, Reichier, & Renner, 1988) administration showed that BK's overall score of 30 placed him in the range of mildly-to-moderately autistic condition. His highest scores (more autistic-like) were in the domains of nonverbal communication, visual response imitation, relating to people, and emotional response. His most appropriate responses were in the domains of object use, listening response, and adaptation to change. Since BK was earlier diagnosed with Tuberous Sclerosis Complex, his autistic condition was considered as syndromic autism, which means it co-exists with a medical condition as a secondary rather than primary disorder of concern (Melillo, 2012).

Second Set of Psycho-educational Assessment Results

In 2011, BK underwent two standardized assessments at the same public hospital when he was first diagnosed with TSC and syndromic autism. The two assessments were (i) Wechsler Adult Intelligence Scale-3rd Edition (WAIS-III); and (ii) the Vineland Adaptive Behavior Scale-2nd Edition (VABS-2). Readers interested to know more about the two standardized assessment tools can refer to Pierangelo and Giuliani (2006) for more detail. The results are briefly described below:

Wechsler Adult Intelligence Scale-3rd Edition (WAIS-3)

The WAIS-3 (Wechsler, 1997) is an individually administered clinical instrument for assessing the intellectual ability of adults aged 16 through 89. BK did not respond to the examiner's questions at the time of assessment. He would repeat single word of the question the examiner posed. Hence, in BK's case, since he was non-verbal, it was impossible to assess him on the complete WAIS-3. Hence, there were no Verbal IQ and Full-Scale IQ could not be computed. The only result available was BK's Performance IQ of 47 at <0.1 percentile rank with 95% confidence interval between 43 and 57. The result indicated BK's extremely low intellectual capacity.

Vineland Adaptive Behavior Scale-2nd Edition (VABS-2)

The focus of VABS-2 (Sparrow, Cicchetti, & Balla, 2005) is to assess the adaptive behaviours of the client, including his ability to cope with environment changes, to learn new everyday skills and demonstrate independence. The primary purpose of the VABS-2 is to assess the social abilities of an individual, whose age ranges from preschool to 90 years. The results reliably reveal crucial information for diagnosing various disabilities, including autism, Asperger syndrome, intellectual disability, and language impairment.

Since the adaptive behaviour is a composite of various dimensions, the VABS-2 covers the following four sub-domains: (i) Communication; (ii) Daily Living Skills; (iii) Socialization; and (iv) Motor Skills; as well as (v) Maladaptive Behaviour, which is optional. Together the v-scores obtained from the four domains a standard score can be obtained for the Adaptive Behaviour Composite (ABC) score.

In BK's VABS-2 results, he scored a low ABC score of 26±7 with <1%ile rank. All his other VABS-2 sub-domains were in the low scores, too: 21±7 for Communication, 46±8 for Daily Living Skills, 23±7 for Socialization, and 47±0 for Motor Skills, all at <1%ile rank.

When comparing the first set of psychoeducational assessment results with the second set, BK's intellectual quotient remained below the standard score of 50 and his adaptive behaviour composite score remained in the low category. According to Meyers, Nihira, and Zetlin (1979) individuals with extremely low levels of cognition, adaptive behaviour tends to fall on par with cognitive ability or mental age. In other words, if cognition is significantly impaired, so are adaptive skills; however, "they tend to be equally impaired" (Saulnier & Klaiman, 2018). Saulnier and Klaiman (2018) argued that this high correlation could be accounted by two main factors: firstly, the limitations in the floor levels of assessment measures for both intellectual capacity (or IQ) and adaptive behaviour; and secondly, it could be due to an overlap in behaviours being assessed at these low levels.

Third Set of Psycho-educational Assessment Results

In 2018, BK's parents sent him to a private assessment and intervention center for a new psychoeducational assessment to be done. It included the following assessments based on the XBA approach: (i) the Stanford-Binet Intelligence Scales-5th Edition (SB-5) (Roid, 2003a); (ii) the Test of Non-verbal Intelligence-3rd Edition (TONI-3) (Brown, Sherbenou, & Johnsen, 1997) (iii) the Sensory Profile-Caregiver Questionnaire (SP-CQ) (Dunn, 1999); (iv) Gilliam Autism Rating Scale (GARS) (Gilliam,1995); (v) the Broad Autism Phenotype Questionnaire (BAPQ) (Hurley et al., 2007); and (vi) the Empathy Quotient (EQ) and Systemizing Quotient (SQ) Questionnaire (EQ-SQQ) (Baron-Cohen et al., 2003). The results from this set of psychoeducational assessment (see Pierangelo & Giuliani, 2006 for detail on the different standardized tests) are presented below:

Stanford-Binet Intelligence Scales-5th Edition (SB-5)

The Stanford-Binet Intelligence Scales-5th Edition (SB-5) (Roid, 2003a) is a wide-ranging, individually administered test battery. Its norms have been designed for age 2 through 85+ years and its subtests cover five cognitive factors: (i) Fluid Reasoning, (ii) Knowledge (i.e., crystallized ability), (iii) Quantitative Reasoning, (iv) Visual-Spatial Processing, and (v) Working Memory – in both verbal (V) and non-verbal (NV) domains.

The SB-5 (Roid, 2003a) was administered to determine BK's intellectual capacity. The SB-5 measures five cognitive abilities in both nonverbal and verbal formats with a total of 10 subtests (Roid, 2003b). Each of these subtests will be described briefly below.

- Fluid Reasoning (FR):
  It measures a student's ability to use inductive or deductive reasoning while solving both verbal and nonverbal problems.
- Knowledge (KN):
  It assesses your child's understanding of general information, vocabulary, social behavioural standards, and common sense that kids within the same age range are also expected to know.
- Quantitative Reasoning (QR):
  It assesses an individual's abilities with basic math concepts (such as identifying numbers and solving math word problems) as well as patterning, sequencing, ordering, classifying, comparing, and numerical problem-solving skills.
- Visual-Spatial Processing (VS):
  It measures each student's ability to identify patterns, relationships, spatial orientations, and how individual pieces relate to whole images on display as well as solve problems using pictures, images, diagrams, geometric shapes, maps or tables.
- Working Memory (WM):
  It assesses a child's ability to access information he or she has just seen or heard and how that data is inspected, transformed or sorted when answering a question or solving problems, such as repeating number and letter sequences in order, tapping blocks in a predetermined pattern or identifying visual and verbal absurdities shown on the test.

Table 5 shows the SB-5 subtests with a brief description of the subtests and their factors.

Table 5. A Brief Description of the SB-5 Subtests (Roid, 2003a)

Fluid Reasoning	Knowledge	Quantitative Reasoning	Visual-Spatial Processing	Working Memory
Early reasoning	Vocabulary	Non-verbal quantitative reasoning (non-verbal)	Form board and form patterns (non-verbal)	Delayed response (non-verbal)
Verbal absurdities	Procedural knowledge (non-verbal)	Verbal quantitative reasoning	Position and direction	Block span (non-verbal)
Verbal analogies	Picture absurdities (non-verbal)			Memory for sentences
Object series matrices (non-verbal)				Last word

BK's SB-5 normed total and subtest scores are shown in two separate tables: Table 2 (Non-Verbal/NV Domain) and Table 3 (Verbal/V Domain).

Table 6 and Table 7 show that both BK's Verbal Intelligence Quotient (VIQ) based on all the five verbal subtests and Non-Verbal Intelligence Quotient (NVIQ) based on all the five non-verbal subtests are in the moderately impaired or delayed intellectual capacity.

Table 6. BK's Non-Verbal (NV) Subtests of SB-5

Subtests	Raw Score	Scaled Score	Standard Score
NV - Fluid Reasoning (NV-FR)	17	1	
NV – Knowledge (NV-KN)	5	1	
NV - Quantitative Reasoning (NV-QR)	3	1	
NV - Visual Spatial (NV-VS)	8	1	
NV – Working Memory (NV-WM)	9	1	
Total Sum of Scores for NVIQ	--	5	42

Table 7. BK's Verbal (V) Subtests of SB-5

Subtests	Raw Score	Scaled Score	Standard Score
V - Fluid Reasoning (V-FR)	2	1	
V – Knowledge (V-KN)	17	1	
V - Quantitative Reasoning (V-QR)	3	1	
V - Visual Spatial (V-VS)	3	1	
V – Working Memory (V-WM)	0	1	
Total Sum of Scores for VIQ	--	5	43

Table 8 shows BK's standard scores for all the combined five non-verbal/verbal (NV/V) subtests in SB-5. His four SB-5 quotients are shown in Table 9.

Table 8. Sum of Scaled Scores for BK's Combined Non-Verbal/Verbal Subtests

Subtests	Sum of Scaled Scores	Percentile Rank	95% Confidence Level
• Fluid Reasoning (FD)	2	<0.1	44-60
• Knowledge (KN)	2	<0.1	45-61
• Quantitative Reasoning (QR)	2	<0.1	46-62
• Visual Spatial (VS)	2	<0.1	44-60
• Working Memory (WM)	2	<0.1	45-61

Table 9. BK's Four SB-5 Quotients[7]

Quotients	Standard Score	Percentile Rank	95% Confidence Interval
NVIQ	42	<0.1	39-51
VIQ	43	<0.1	39-51
FSIQ	30	<0.1	37-45
AbIQ	47	<0.1	44-60

Each of the four SB-5 quotients (Roid, 2003a, 2003b) is briefly explained as follows:

- Non-Verbal Intelligence Quotient (NVIQ):
  This is the normed combined score taken from the five non-verbal subtests.
- Verbal Intelligence Quotient (VIQ):
  This is the normed combined score taken from the five verbal subtests.
- Full Scale Intelligence Quotient (FSIQ):
  This is the normed combined score taken from all 10 non-verbal and verbal subtests.
- Abbreviated Battery IQ (AbIQ):
  This is computed to provide a quick estimate of two major cognitive factors: fluid reasoning and crystallized ability.

As shown in Table 9 above, BK's SB-5 NVIQ-VIQ profile shows that his NVIQ is equivalent to VIQ (i.e., NVIQ $\equiv$ VIQ) by a difference of 1 point. The minimum SB-5 NVIQ-VIQ difference of 9-10 points is required for significance at the .05 level (Roid, 2003b). His NVIQ-VIQ profile is typical of individuals with extremely low intelligence i.e., he has intellectual and developmental disorder (Roid & Barram, 2004).

A combination of the standard scores from both NVIQ and VIQ was used to compute the FSIQ. BK's FSIQ is 40. Since BK's FSIQ is less than 70, it indicates that he shows moderately impaired or delayed verbal and non-verbal skills.

During the SB-5 administration, BK displayed short attention-concentration span that interfered with the testing procedure. Hence, AbIQ, which offers a more valid estimate of BK's true intelligence, was computed as it is more representative of the full battery for him. The AbIQ is used here as its short administration time helps to minimize off-tasks behaviour and maximize attention (Roid, 2003b). BK's AbIQ is 47. However, care should be taken when interpreting the AbIQ as it may overestimate true abilities (Roid & Barram, 2004). BK's FSIQ < AbIQ by a difference of 7 points. The minimum difference required for significance at the .05 level is 10-11 points as outlined in the SB-5 Test Manual (Roid, 2003b).

BK's AbIQ of 47 coincided exactly with his previous Performance IQ of 47 based on WAIS- III administration. His NVIQ based on SB-5 administration is 42, one point lower than his VIQ. His Full-Scale IQ based on SB-5 administration is 40. All the standard scores are in the moderately impaired or delayed range (40 to 54). The SB-5 IQ range (deviation IQ) and the IQ classification (descriptors for the nine ranges) are shown in Table 10 below.

---

[7] Abbreviations for Non-Verbal Intelligence Quotient (NVIQ), Verbal Intelligence Quotient (VIQ), Full Scale Intelligence Quotient (FSIQ) and Abbreviated Battery Intelligence Quotient (AbIQ) will be used throughout this paper.

Table 10. Description and Classification of the SB-5 IQ Range

IQ Range ("deviation IQ")	IQ Classification
145-160	Very gifted or highly advanced
130-144	Gifted or very advanced
120-129	Superior
110-119	High average
90-109	Average
80-89	Low average
70-79	Borderline impaired or delayed
55-69	Mildly impaired or delayed
40-54	Moderately impaired or delayed

Summary of Findings from SB-5 Administration

In BK's case, his V-IQ was 43 and his NV-IQ was 42, both at <0.1%ile rank and in the range 39-51 at 95% confidence interval. His Full-Scale IQ was 30 within the severely retarded range of 20-34 (Cooijmans, 2003). BK's NV-IQ/V-IQ profile showed that his NV-IQ was equivalent to V-IQ (i.e., NVIQ=VIQ) with only a difference by 1 point. The minimum NV-IQ/V-IQ difference of 9-10 points is required for significance at the .05 level (Roid, 2003b). BK's NV-IQ/V-IQ profile at the time of assessment was typical of individuals with extremely low intelligence. In other words, based on his SB-5 results, BK was diagnosed with intellectual and developmental disorder (Roid and Barram, 2004). A combination of the standard scores from both NV-IQ and V-IQ was used to compute the FSIQ. BK's FSIQ was 30. Since BK's FSIQ was less than 70, it indicated that he had severely impaired or delayed verbal and non-verbal skills.

During the SB-5 administration, BK also observed to have a short attention-concentration span that interfered with the testing procedure. Hence, Abbreviated Battery IQ (AbIQ), which offers a more valid estimate of BK's true intelligence, was computed as it would be more representative of the full SB-5 battery for him. The AbIQ was used in this case as its short administration time could help to minimize off-tasks behaviour and maximize attention (Roid, 2003b). BK's AbIQ was 47. However, care should be taken when interpreting the AbIQ as it may overestimate true abilities (Roid and Barram, 2004). BK's FSIQ<AbIQ by a difference of 7 points. The minimum difference required for significance at the .05 level is 10-11 points as outlined in the SB-5 Test Manual (Roid, 2003b). BK's AbIQ of 47 (at <0.1%ile rank; 95% confidence interval within the range of 44-60) coincided exactly with his previous Performance IQ of 47 based on the WAIS-3 administration. His NV-IQ based on the SB-5 administration was 42, just one point lower than V-IQ. His Full-Scale IQ based on the SB-5 administration was 40 (at <0.1%ile rank; 95% confidence level in the range of 37 and 45). All the standard scores were in the moderately impaired or delayed range (40-54) (Cooijmans, 2003).

Test of Non-Verbal Intelligence-3rd Edition (TONI-3)

The Test of Nonverbal Intelligence-3rd Edition (TONI-3; Brown, Sherbenou, and Johnsen, 1997) is designed to test non-verbal abstract/figural problem solving in several content areas: shape, position, direction, rotation, contiguity, shading, size and movement. It was administered to determine BK's non-verbal problem-solving ability in term of his deviation quotient.

The SB-5 results (see Tables 2, 3, 4 and 5 above) have indicated clearly that BK has intellectual impairment. The TONI-3 was administered to determine BK's non-verbal problem-solving ability in term of his deviation quotient. The TONI-3 results (see Table 7) show that BK's performance in the test was less than 70, which means his NVIQ is in the very poor range.

Table 11 shows BK's deviation quotient is 64 (very poor) with an equivalent age of 5 years

9 months as compared with his current chronological age of 31 years 1 month. The Deviation Quotient (NV) of 64 places BK in the mildly impaired or delayed range of nonverbal cognitive ability. This non-verbal standard score based on the TONI-3 administration is one level higher than the results of the standard scores based on the SB-5 administration.

Table 11. BK's TONI-3 Scores

ONI-3 Scores	Scores	Age Equivalent	Descriptor
Deviation Quotient	64	--	Very poor
Standard Error of Measurement (SEM)	4	--	--
Percentile Rank	< 1	--	--
Total Raw Score	4	--	--
Age Equivalent	4	5 years 9 months	Extremely impaired

Summary of Findings from TONI-3 Administration

BK's deviation quotient or NVIQ of 64 ((at <1%ile rank; SEM=4); very poor) with an equivalent age of 5 years 9 months as compared with his chronological age of 31 years at the time of assessment put him in the mildly impaired or delayed range of nonverbal cognitive ability. This nonverbal standard score based on the TONI-3 administration is one level higher than the results of the standard scores based on the SB-5 administration.

Kellogg Scribbles Test

Back in 1994, BK was said to be able to accurately draw vertical and horizontal lines in the Beery-Buktenica Developmental Test of Visual-Motor Integration (Beery, 1997). However, in 2018, when BK was asked to draw a person, he could only produce scribbles (e.g., dot, single or multiple vertical lines, single or multiple horizontal lines) on the paper at the time of assessment. According to Kellogg (1970) the vertical and horizontal lines are two out of 20 basic scribbles that constitute "the building blocks of art, and they are important because they permit a detailed and comprehensive description of the work of young preschool children" (p.15). The Table 12 below lists all the 20 basic scribbles:

Table 12. The 20 Basic Scribbles

Basic Scribble	Scribble Descriptor	Basic Scribble	Scribble Descriptor
Type 1	Dot	Type 11	Roving enclosing line
Type 2	Single vertical line	Type 12	Zigzag or waving line
Type 3	Single horizontal line	Type 13	Single loop line
Type 4	Single diagonal line	Type 14	Multiple loop line
Type 5	Single curved line	Type 15	Spiral line
Type 6	Multiple vertical line	Type 16	Multiple-line overlaid circle
Type 7	Multiple horizontal line	Type 17	Multiple-line circumference circle
Type 8	Multiple diagonal line	Type 18	Circular line spread out
Type 9	Multiple curved line	Type 19	Single crossed circle
Type 10	Roving open line	Type 20	Imperfect circle

Source: Kellogg (1970).

Sensory Profile-Caregiver Questionnaire (SP-CQ)

The Sensory Profile-Caregiver Questionnaire (SP-CQ; Dunn, 1999) was completed by BK's mother as BK was not cognitively capable of completing the Sensory Profile Self-Questionnaire himself (as reported by Camulli, Goh, & Chia, 2018). The aim of profile was to ascertain if Benjamin displayed any sensory-related processing, modulation and/or emotional-behavioural problems that could have interfered with his thinking/learning. Moreover, it was also to find out Benjamin's SP factors as well as the Sensory Profile summary of his sensory processing, modulation, behaviour and emotional responses to external/internal stimuli.

The SP-CQ (Dunn, 1999), the caregiver's version of questionnaire (by proxy), was completed by BK's mother as BK is not cognitively capable of completing the Sensory Profile Self-Questionnaire. The aim of profile is to ascertain if BK has any sensory-related processing, modulation and/or emotional-behavioural problems that could have interfered with his thinking/learning. Moreover, it is also to find out BK's Sensory Profile factors (see Table 8) as well as the Sensory Profile summary of his sensory processing, modulation, and behaviour and emotional responses to external/internal stimuli (see Table 8).

Table 13 highlights two areas of concern regarding (1) low endurance/tone and (2) sedentary about BK. According to Whitney (2016), low endurance/tone means "the lack of supportive muscle tone, usually with increased mobility at the joints; the person with low tone has limbs that are floppy, appear to not be attached to the body, and have awkward movement patterns. This lack of muscle tone results in poor ability to act in a sustained state of alert performance" (para. 18).

Table 13. BK's Performance in the Sensory Profile (Caregiver Version) Factor Scores

Factor	Factor Raw Score Total	Typical Performance	Probable Difference	Definite Difference
• Sensory Seeking	70/85	√		
• Emotionally Reactive	65/80	√		
• Low Endurance/Tone	22/45			√
• Oral Sensory Sensitivity	30/45		√	
• Inattention/Distractibility	24/35		√	
• Poor Registration	30/40		√	
• Sensory Sensitivity	14/20		√	
• Sedentary	8/20			√
• Fine Motor/Perceptual	10/15	√		

Table 14 (i.e., 14a, 14b and 14c) shows those sensory areas where BK is still exhibiting definite issues of concern, especially in these three main Sensory Profile (Dunn, 1999) areas: (1) sensory processing related to endurance/tone; (2) modulation of sensory input affecting emotional responses; and (3) behavioural outcomes of sensory processing.

Table 14a. BK's Raw Scores in the Area of the Sensory Processing of the Sensory Profile

Sensory Processing	Section Raw Score Total	Typical Performance	Probable Difference	Definite Difference
Auditory Processing	30/40	√		
Visual Processing	36/45	√		
Vestibular Processing	45/55		√	
Touch Processing	65/90		√	
Multisensory Processing	27/35	√		
Oral Sensory Processing	45/60		√	

Table 14b. BK's Raw Scores in the Area of the Sensory Modulation of the Sensory Profile

Sensory Modulation	Section Raw Score Total	Typical Performance	Probable Difference	Definite Difference
Sensory Processing related to Endurance/Tone	22/45			√
Modulation related to Body Position & Movement	41/50	√		
Modulation of Movement affecting Activity Level	19/35		√	
Modulation of Sensory Input affecting Emotional Response	11/20			√
Modulation of Visual Input affecting Emotional Response & Activity Level	12/20		√	

Table 14c. BK's Raw Scores in the Behaviour and Emotional Responses of the Sensory Profile

Behaviour & Emotional Responses	Section Raw Score Total	Typical Performance	Probable Difference	Definite Difference
Emotional/Social Responses	68/85	√		
Behavioural Outcomes of Sensory Processing	18/30			√
Items indicating Thresholds for Response	10/15		√	

Summary of Findings from SP-CQ Administration

There were two areas of concern for BK: (i) low endurance/tone, i.e., BK would prefer to be a bystander than a participator; and (ii) sedentary (i.e., a strong preference to be left alone). According to Whitney (2016) low endurance/tone means "lack of supportive muscle tone, usually with increased mobility at the joints; the person with low tone has limbs that are floppy, appear to not be attached to the body, and have awkward movement patterns. This lack of muscle tone results in poor ability to act in a sustained state of alert performance" (para.18).

Gilliam Autism Rating Scale (GARS)

The Gilliam Autism Rating Scale (GARS; Gilliam,1995) is an individually-administered, norm-referenced screening measure designed in a rating scale-format. Its purpose is to identify individuals suspected with autism as well as other severe behavioural problems. The GARS measure provides an overall score known as Autism Quotient (AQ), which is computed from three or four subscales: (1) Stereotyped Behaviours; (2) Communication; (3) Social interaction; and/or (4) Developmental Disturbance.

From the GARS administration, BK's AQ of 102 is 12 points above 90. This indicates that he is probably autistic. The scaled scores of 8 through 12 or AQ of 90 through 110 are within the average range for an individual with autism in the normative sample. According to Gilliam (1995), "[A]pproximately 50% of the subjects with autism scored in this range" (p. 17).

BK's Autism Quotient (AQ) of 102 is above 90, as shown in Table 15. He is probably autistic. Scaled score of 8 through 12 or AQ of 90 through 110 are within the average range for an individual with autism in the normative sample. "Approximately 50% of the subjects with autism scored in this range" (Gilliam, 1995, p.17).

Table 15. BK's Gilliam Autism Rating Scale (GARS) Scores

Subtests	Raw Score	Scaled Scores	Percentile Rank	SEM
Stereotyped Behaviours	19	10	50	1
Communication	29	13	84	1
Social Interaction	20	8	25	1
Developmental Disturbances	6	10	50	1
Sum of Scaled Scores	--	41	--	--
Autism Quotient (AQ)	--	102	55	3
Probability of Autism	Average			

Summary of Findings from GARS Administration

From the GARS administration, BK's scaled scores for the four subscales were 10, 13, 8 and 10, respectively. Though all the four scaled scores were in the average range, BK performed worst in the social interaction subtest with a subscale score of 8.

With an AQ of 102, i.e., 12 points above 90, this indicated that BK's condition included the high probability of autism (Camulli, Goh, & Chia, 2018). According to Jeste et al. (2014) TSC "confers a high risk of autism spectrum disorders (ASDs) and intellectual disability, with rates of ASD ranging from 25% to 60%, much higher than the 1% to 2% reported in the general population" (p.160). On the reverse, Gillberg and Coleman (1996) reported an estimated 9% of children with autistic disorder have TSC. In other words, it is more common for children with TSC to have a syndromic autism than children with ASD to have tuberous sclerosis. The scaled scores of 8 through 12 or AQ of 90 through 110 on the GARS are within the average range of an individual with autism in the normative sample. According to Gilliam (1995) "Approximately 50% of the subjects with autism scored in this range" (p.17).

Broad Autism Phenotype Questionnaire (BAPQ)

The BAPQ (Hurley et al., 2007) is used to find out about a set personality and language characteristics that reflect the phenotypic expression of the genetic liability to autism, in non-autistic relatives of autistic individuals. The BAPQ includes both self-and informant-report versions. It consists of "three subscales corresponding to the triad of characteristics associated with the primary diagnostic domains of autism: (1) social abnormalities, (2) pragmatic language difficulties and (3) rigid personality and a desire of sameness" (Sasson et al., 2013).

However, in BK's case, his parents did not complete the BAPQ for reasons unknown and hence, the questionnaire was aborted or could not be used for analysis because most items were not completed (as reported by Camulli, Goh, & Chia, 2018).

Empathy Quotient-Systemizing Quotient Questionnaire for Adults

The Empathy Quotient (EQ) and Systemizing Quotient (SQ) Questionnaire (EQ-SQQ) was developed in order to examine trends in gender typical behaviour in adults (Baron-Cohen et al., 2003; Baron-Cohen & Wheelwright 2004; Wheelwright et al., 2006). The EQ-SQQ constitutes both EQ and SQ self-report questionnaires with a Likert format and contain a list of statements about real life situations, experiences and interests where empathizing or systemizing skills are required.

The questionnaire was done by BK's mother (by proxy) since BK is unable to understand the items stated in it. Like the BAP Questionnaire, it was also aborted or could not be used for analysis because most items were not completed (as reported by Camulli, Goh, & Chia, 2018).

Comparison of the Three Sets of Psychoeducational Assessment Results

When comparing the third set of psychoeducational assessment results with the first and second sets, as reported by Goh and Xie (2019) as well as Camulli, Goh and Chia (2018) in their respective papers, BK's intellectual quotient based on the SB-5 administration for both V-IQ of 43 and NV-IQ of 42 remained below the standard score of 50, but his NVIQ of 64 based on the TONI-3 administration put him in the category of mild intellectual disability. There was no adaptive behaviour measure (e.g., Vineland Adaptive Behavior Scale-2nd Edition and/or Adaptive Behavior Diagnostic Scale) done in the third set of psychoeducational assessment. Hence, there was no way to compare if cognition could be significantly more impaired than adaptive skills. BK's AQ of 102 also put in the range of high probability of autism. As mentioned earlier, "[A]pproximately 50% of the subjects in the normative sample with autism scored in this range" (Gilliam, 1995). BK's SP-CQ results indicated that he was very much a sedentary bystander than an engaging participator.

In summarizing the psychoeducational diagnosis for BK, he was a young adult diagnosed with TSC and had a comorbid condition of severely low-functioning (IQ below 50) non-verbal (lacking speech) syndromic (not primary disorder as it coexists with TSC) autistic crypto-savant (hidden talent) disorder (LF-NV-SACSD) or low-functioning non-verbal autistic crypto-savantism (LF-NV-ACS). Camulli and Goh (2018) used the term autistic savant spectrum syndromic disorder (ASSSD) to describe BK's condition. Table 16 provides a summary of the findings:

Table 16. A Summary of the Psycho-educational Assessment Results

Assessment Factors	1st Psychoeducational assessment	2nd Psychoeducational assessment	3rd Psychoeducational assessment
Year of Assessment	1997	2011	2018
Intellectual Quotient	IQ <50 (LIPS-R)	PIQ=47 (WAIS-3)	V-IQ=43 (SB-5) NV-IQ=42 (SB-5) FSIQ=30 (SB-5) AbIQ=47 (SB-5)
Sensory Pattern	Not available	Not available	Low Endurance/Tone (SP-CQ) Sedentary (SP-CQ)
Adaptive Behaviour Quotient	ABC=Low (VABS-I)	ABC=26$\pm$7 (VABS-2) Com=21$\pm$7 (VAB-2) ADL=46$\pm$8 (VABS-2) Soc=23$\pm$7 (VABS-2) Motor=47$\pm$0 (VABS-2)	Not available
Autistic Quotient:	Mild-to-moderate autistic spectrum condition (CARS)	Not available	AQ=102 (GARS) SB=10 (GARS) Com=13 (GARS) SI=8 (GARS) DD=10 (GARS) Mild-to-moderate autism
Concluding remarks:	Severe intellectual disability with mild-to-moderate autism	Severe intellectual disability with low adaptive behaviour skills	Severe intellectual disability with poor sensory processing and mild-to-moderate autism

The abovementioned assessment results agree to one common psychoeducational diagnosis – in addition to BK's TSC condition – of his severe intellectual disability and mild/moderate autism.

Post-Assessment Discussion

When BK was younger, he "possessed an innate ability to play piano by just listening to the tune without being taught and had even performed at a performance concert" (Camulli & Goh, 2018). His parents did not realize his savant talent and hired a piano teacher to teach him according to her method. This caused BK to be resistant and soon he lost his interest in piano playing. "Almost as soon as his musical talent was discovered, this savant ability was lost immediately. It was a clear indication of BK's early innate ability without teaching or training" (Camulli & Goh, 2018).

Several years later, BK developed a keen interest in painting, which was only noticed in 2014, when he participated in a church event to paint a mural on the side of the church car park. BK's earlier two sets of assessment results done in 1991 and 2011 indicated his severe intellectual impairment along with syndromic autism as well as all his medical diagnosis, TSC, yet, BK exhibited a special talent in painting (as well as piano playing).

An art teacher was hired to teach him. However, there was not much the art teacher could do except to facilitate and go along with BK's interest. All that could be done was to provide him with necessary tools and materials. Since then, it has become evident that BK does possess a strong systemizing ability or special talent in painting. Every piece is painted with loads of patience and more patience. It is a long process, and Camulli and Goh (2018) have described this as a manifestation of a savant artist, BK. Being identified as a savant artist, BK met the following savant traits listed by Treffert (2010):

(i)   An underlying disability: BK has been diagnosed to have TSC with ID and syndromic autism as well as savant syndrome;

(ii) An innate ability without teaching or training: BK paints without formal lessons but an art teacher was hired to facilitate his painting activities;

(iii) A talent which typically 'explodes' on the scene at a very early age, but BK's gift of painting was not known until he was an adult in his twenties. Camulli and Goh (2018) who have worked with BK before, disagreed with Treffert (2010) on this trait. They argued that very severely disabled do not exhibit their own talents which are masked, suppressed or hidden by their severe or profound disabilities;

(iv) An obsessive preoccupation with the skill: BK has an obsessive habit of picking up tiny circular items found on the ground anywhere which may not seem to be related to what savant is known for. "However, it can be regarded as an essential pre-skill that is very much required in being observant for the fine details in drawing or painting" (Camulli and Goh, 2018);

(v)   A prolific output of product on a continuous basis: BK continues to demonstrate "a prolific output of product (i.e., paintings) on a continuous basis" (Camulli and Goh, 2018) over the years and has also held exhibitions for his paintings, many of which have been sold; and

(vi) A literal, eidetic-like memory with massive capacity in the area of expertise: BK possesses such a memory. For example, BK could recall the exact route his parents and/or he had taken before a long time ago, even if that had happened once, and he knew when a wrong turn was made.

All the six savant traits put forth by Treffert (2010) are re-categorized under the following three core symptoms by Camulli and Goh (2018) (see Table 17 below):

Table 17. The Three Core Symptoms of Savantism

Symptoms	First Core Symptom	Second Core Symptom	Third Core Symptom
Descriptors	Presence of an underlying disability	One or more of the underlying superior systemizing abilities (Myers, Baron-Cohen, and Wheelwright, 2004)	Over-excitability in one, two or more areas of extreme interests (see Chia and Lim, 2017; Dabrowski, 1972, for detail).
Examples	TSC, hyperlexia, Heller 's Syndrome, etc.	Motoric, mechanical, abstract, social, natural, and organizable	Psychomotor, sensual, intellectual, emotional, and imaginational
Traits based on Treffert's (2010) categories	Trait #1	Traits #2, #3 and #6	Traits #4 and #5

It is the second core symptom that the authors of this monograph have taken an interest to explore further in terms of the formulation of systemizing by Baron-Cohen (2006) in the following cognitive process: [input]→[operation]→[output]. To understand this 3-step process, the term *system* must first be understood. Baron-Cohen et al. (2003) defined a system as "something that takes inputs, which can then be operated on in variable ways, to deliver different outputs in a rule-governed way" (p.1). Generally, as already briefly described earlier, there are at least six kinds of system: (i) abstract (e.g., multiplication/repeated addition), (ii) motoric (e.g., steps involved in butterfly stroke technique in swimming), (iii) natural (e.g., soil erosion on a hillside after a thunderstorm), (iv) organizable (e.g., arranging books according to height), (v) social (e.g., a family tree or genogram), and (vi) technical (e.g., operating an electric drill). All these six systems share the same underlying process, which can be observed during systemizing: INPUT → OPERATION → OUTPUT.

Using the 3-step cognitive process, Goh and Xie (2019) examined BK's painting talent in terms of his systemizing ability in painting. BK has since produced many paintings – many of them have been sold at local arts exhibitions – and that goes to show he has an eye for detail, colour texture, and stroke application (see Figure 11 to 14 below).

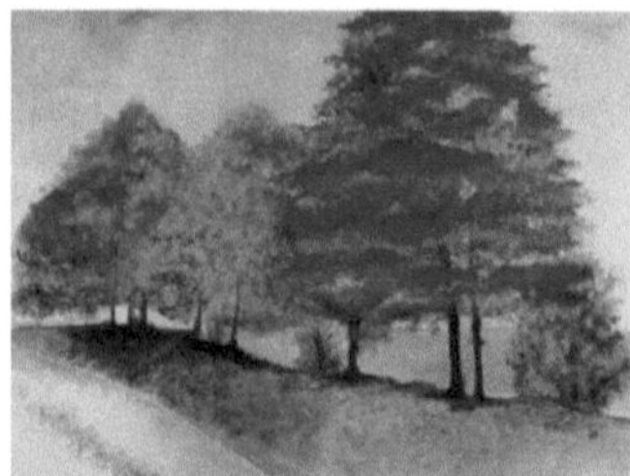

Figure 11. Trees in Autumn.

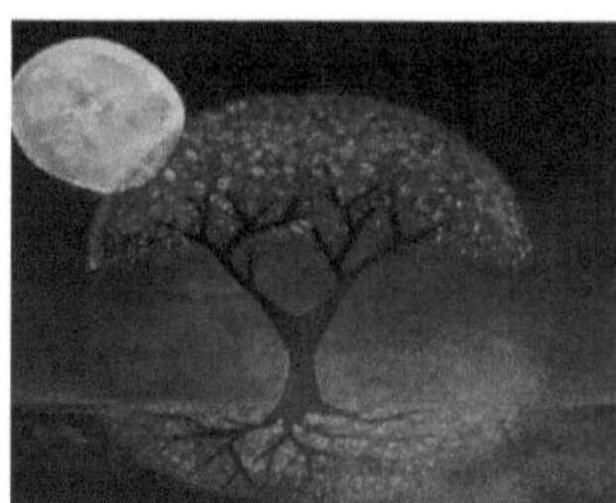

Figure 12. A Tree under the Moon.

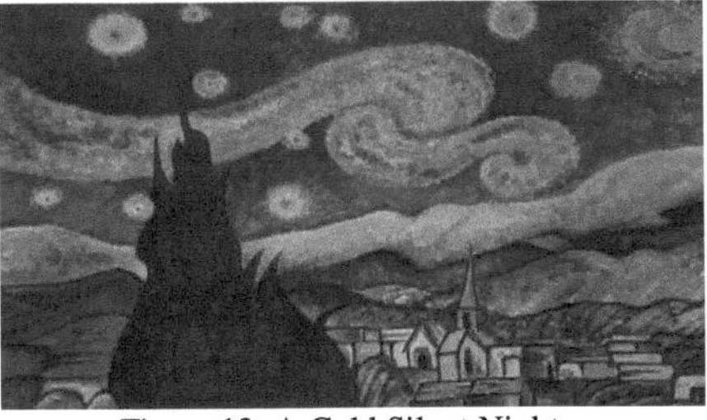

Figure 13. A Cold Silent Night.

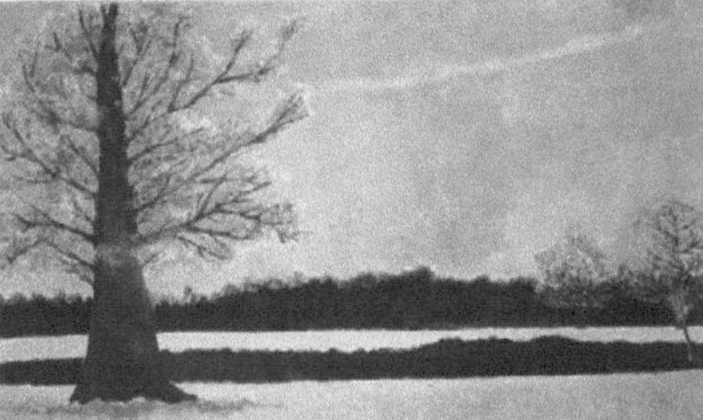

Figure 14. A Tree in Winter.

Despite his current medical conditions (i.e., TSC, ID and ASD), BK has been endowed with the ability to create by his special talent in painting (Goh & Xie, 2019). According to Simons (2004) a successful painting (using acrylics and oils) involves seven steps that constitute this specific systemizing ability as reported by Goh and Xie (2019, pp.24-25):

(1) See with an observant eye for the subject to be drawn/painted;

(2) Under-paint the canvas to eliminate "the harsh, intimidating white canvas" and allow the freedom to paint in whatever way that pleases the artist;

(3) Identify the big shapes in order to organize the composition of the painting over the surface of the canvas (see Figure 15 below);

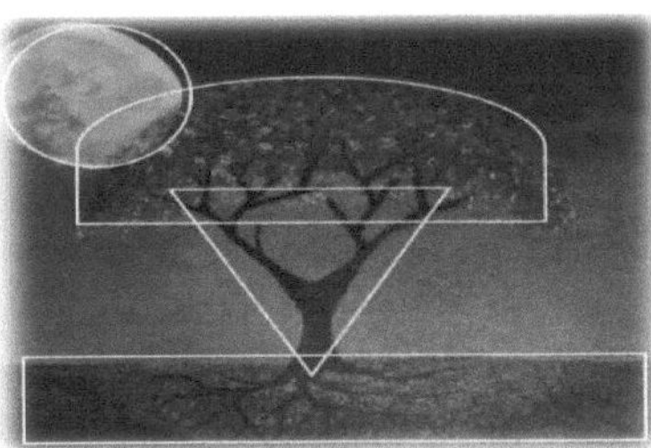

Figure 15. BK's Recognition of the Big Shapes for the Composition of His Painting

(4) Squint at the image that has been drawn/painted without having to see the colour. In other words, "work through a value study" (Simons, 2004) i.e., starting with darkest dark and working through about five values, to the lightest (see Figure 16a, 16b and 16c below);

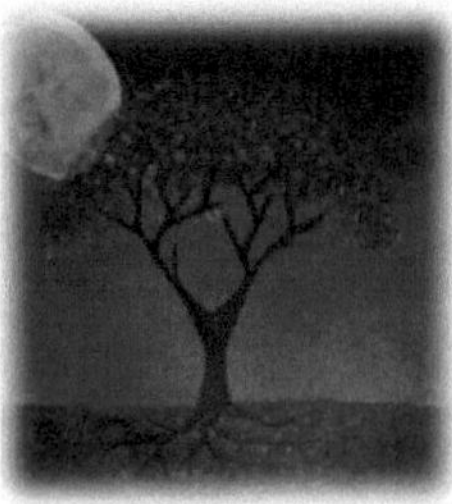
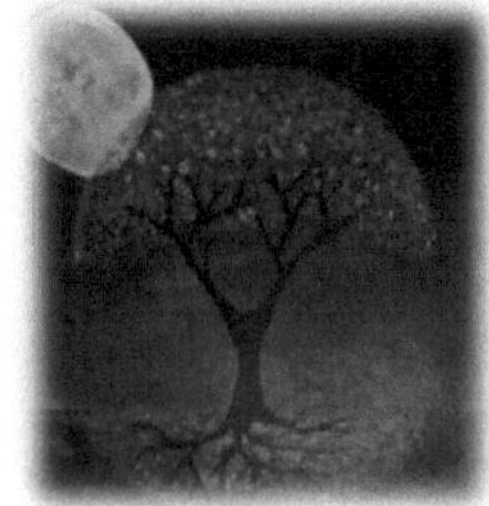
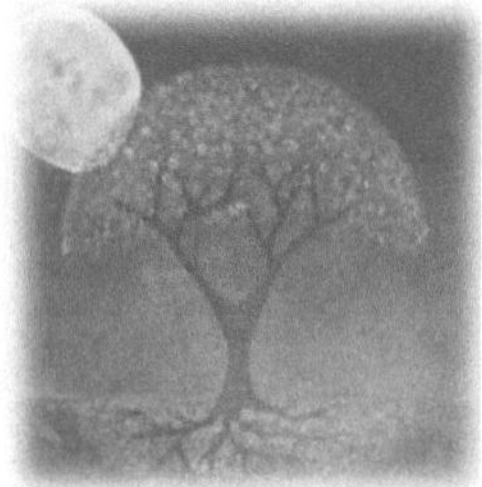

Figure 16a	Figure 16b	Figure16c

Figure 16. An Example of 3-Value Study using BK's painting of "A Tree under the Moon".

(5) Block the colours in the painting, i.e., each colour that is "put on must be same value as what is underneath it, otherwise the painting will 'collapse'!" (Simons, 2004)
(6) Adjust colour and value to "make them (colours) sing" … "Let the paint be paint – don't force it to be a tree or a flower. It has beauty in itself" (Simons, 2004); and
(7) Finish the painting, but '[R]esist the temptation to fix everything … a good time to put on a few highlights with thick paint in the lightest areas – ever so gently lay the paint on top in one stroke without scrubbing" (Simons, 2004). The final product is shown in Figure 17 below.

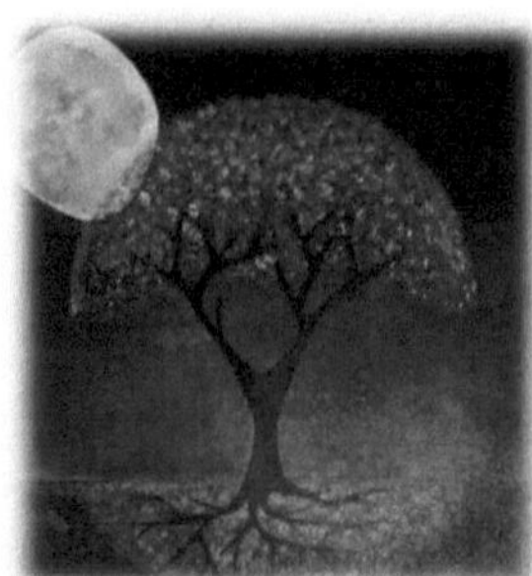

Figure 17. BK's Final Product of His Painting.

Goh and Chia (2019) broke down the above 7-step procedure of painting as proposed by Simons (2004) into the 3-step cognitive process of systemizing: the input→operation→output process can be presented as follows (see Figure 18 below):

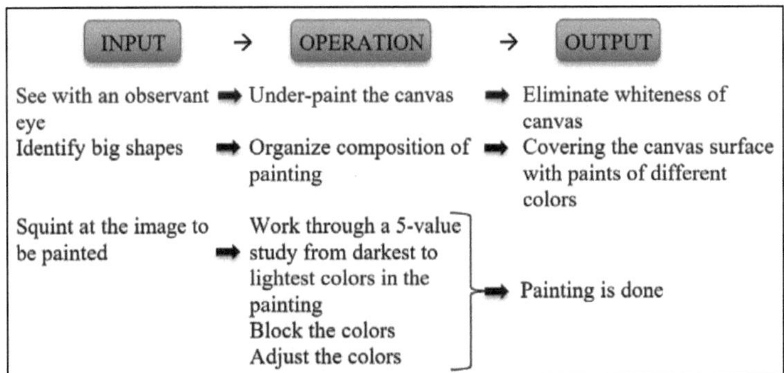

Figure 18. The Systemizing Process of Painting.

BK sees images on the internet with an observant eye and produces replicas of them through his paintings. Over a period of time, he has begun including or omitting images according to what he likes or dislikes and this habit has persisted even today, as shown in his painting. According to Camulli and Goh (2018) BK's "paintings have begun to show more interpretation in the recent months, resulting in more personalized results in his paintings" (p.199). Gradually, BK's interpretation – free form style or some other forms of creativity – is expressed in his fresh, original work (Hosseini, 2012): a truly remarkable ability of a crypto-savant artist, BK's talent (despite his TSC condition with comorbid severe ID and LF/NVASD) via his systemizing ability in acrylic painting has come to light because of his/her syndromic autistic savantism.

CHAPTER FOUR
THE PROOF OF AN ADULT SAVANT ARTIST

In the previous chapters, much has been said about BK, who has been diagnosed with Tuberous Sclerosis Complex (TSC) with syndromic autism (see Camulli, Goh, & Chia, 2018, for detail). In this chapter, the focus is on showing that BK is indeed a savant artist by re-examining his case and to state our points why we strongly believe he is a savant artist.

Core Symptom of Underlying Disability

This core symptom relates to Treffertian trait #1. BK is diagnosed having TSC by medical specialists both in Singapore and overseas (see medical reports provided by his parents) with autistic spectrum conditions (ASC) (based on CARS results). According to Tuberous Sclerosis Alliance (2018), 50% of individuals with TSC are also diagnosable with autism. As many as 14% of individuals with ASD and seizure disorder may also be diagnosable with TSC. Researchers aren't completely sure why ASD and TSC seem to be connected, but according to the Tuberous Sclerosis Alliance (2018), the recent finding suggests that in TSC: "... there are abnormalities in the way different parts of the brain connect to each other, not only in the temporal lobes but in many other parts of the brain as well. These abnormal connections, which occur independent of tubers, are associated with ASD in children and adults with TSC. Additionally, many studies have shown that seizures and, particularly, early onset of seizures, are associated with delayed development and ASD. Therefore, it is likely a combination of factors that leads to the much higher chance of ASD." (para. 3-4).

In addition, results from the Wechsler Adult Intelligence Scales (WAIS-3) could only say that BK's Performance IQ (PIQ) was 47. His latest IQ test done in 2017 suggested that his Non-verbal IQ (NVIQ) = 42 and his Verbal IQ (VIQ) = 43. His fluid reasoning, knowledge, quantitative reasoning, visual-spatial perception, and working memory are less than 0.1 percentile rank. His Abbreviated Battery IQ based on Stanford-Binet 5th Edition (SB-5) = 47, which measures fluid reasoning and crystallized ability. His NVIQ of 64 placed him in the range of extremely impaired.

Despite having extremely impaired intellectual capacity, BK could still produce such wonderful painting with some basic facilitation, guidance and support.

Core Symptom of One/More Underlying Superior Systemising Abilities

This core symptom consists of three Treffertian traits #2, 3 and 6, i.e., innate abilities without teaching or training, talent which typically 'explodes' on the scene at a very early age, and literal, eidetic-like memory with massive capacity in the area of expertise, respectively.

BK, at his younger age, possessed an innate ability to play piano by just listening to the tune without being taught and had even performed at a performance concert. However, his parents did not realise this savant talent and hired a piano teacher to teach him, according to her method. It only caused BK to become resistant and lose his interest in music and especially in piano playing. Almost as soon as his musical talent was discovered, this savant ability was lost quickly. This is a clear indication of BK's early innate ability without teaching or training. Later, he had to be coached to take up another interest of his choice ... it so happened painting came into the picture. It began with a wall mural painting in the church that his talent was discovered. BK kept telling his mother "paint, paint" and an art teacher was hired to teach him. This is very typical of Singaporean parents' expectation: if a child wants to learn music, get a music teacher or send him/her for music class; if the child wants to draw and/or paint, get an art teacher or send him/her for art class; if the child wants to write, send him/her to attend a creative writing class. In fact, there is not much the art teacher could do except to facilitate and go along with BK's interest, e.g., he saw the blood moon and wanted to paint it, and all that could be done was to provide him with the necessary tools and materials.

Among the tests done on BK, his VABS (Vineland Adaptive Behaviour Scales) results showed that his overall adaptive behaviour composite or level is low with a standard score of 26 ± 7 (at 95% confidence level) which is less than 1 percentile rank. Among all the VABS subdomains, i.e., Communication[8], Daily Living Skills[9], Socialisation[10], and Motor Skills, BK's highest standard score of 47 ± 0 (at 95% confidence level), which is less than 1 percentile rank and low adaptive level is his performance in Motor Skills. According to BK's VABS report, his motor/perceptual skills have been estimated to be the best among the four adaptive behaviour subdomains.

According to the Treffertian trait #3, a savant's talent typically 'explodes' on the scene at a very early age. However, we beg to disagree with this trait. Not all savants, and especially crypto-savants, suddenly 'explode' their talents at a very early age. Those who are very severely handicapped or disabled do not exhibit such talents clearly because their talents would be masked, suppressed or hidden by their severe or profound disabilities. For example, YY is one such example of an autistic crypto-savant and it is only in 2017 that his talent was "discovered" at the age of 13 years old and the Very Special Arts (VSA) – a non-government organisation that caters to the artistic needs of individuals with special needs in Singapore – took him up only much later in that same year (see Lim & Chia, 2017, for detail).

In an art book highlighting the talents of several autistic savant artists titled "The Art of Autism: Shifting Perceptions" (Hosseini, 2013), Treffert dispels commonly held misconceptions about autistic savant artists and reminds us that "The remarkable abilities of the artist surface because of their autism, not in spite of it." (p. 30-31). The works celebrated in this book profile artists who began to exhibit their talent and practice their skill at varying ages, from 3 years old to twenty years of age.

For this specific issue of "exploded talent", we would further argue that it depends on the time of onset in the same way not all individuals develop in the same way or same time or at the same developmental pace. It is also important to take note that to understand savant or crypto-savant abilities, we need to understand also gifted/talented abilities. According to the National Association for Gifted Children, "Gifted individuals are those who demonstrate outstanding levels of aptitude (defined as an exceptional ability to reason and learn) or competence (documented performance or achievement in top 10% or rarer) in one or more domains. Domains include any structured area of activity with its own symbol system (e.g., mathematics, music, language) and/or set of sensorimotor skills (e.g., painting, dance, sports)" (para. 5). According to Betts and Niehart (1988), there are six types of gifted individuals[11]: the successful, the challenging, the underground,

---

[8] Communication: standard score of 21 ± 7 (95% conf. level) at <1%ile rank with low adaptive level.

[9] Daily Living Skills: standard score of 46 ± 8 (95% conf. level) at <1%ile rank with low adaptive level; second highest score after Motor Skills.

[10] Socialisation: standard score of 23 ± 7 (95% conf. level) at <1%ile rank with low adaptive level.

[11] Type 1-The Successful Gifted: They display appropriate behaviour, learn well, able to score high on achievement tests and tests of intelligence and seldom manifest problematic behavior because they are eager for approval from the adults (e.g., teachers and parents).
Type 2-The Challenging Gifted: They possess a high degree of creativity, may appear to be stubborn, tactless, or sarcastic, do not conform to the system, and hence, are often at odds with the authority, be it in school or at home.
Type 3-The Underground Gifted: They hide their giftedness and deny their talent in order to feel more included with a non-gifted peer group. They frequently feel insecure and anxious.

the dropout, the double-labelled (also known as the twice-exceptional), and the autonomous. Most of the successful and autonomous gifted individuals can be easily identified by their overt competence. However, the challenging, the underground, the dropout and the double-labelled gifted individuals are the ones whose giftedness is masked or hidden (covert competence) from the adults (e.g., teachers and parents) as well as their peers. Similarly, for the savants and crypto-savants, although they exhibit very poor intellectual capacity (aptitude), their high competence in certain very specific skills in one or more domains can be either overt (savants) or covert (crypto-savants) (see Figure 19).

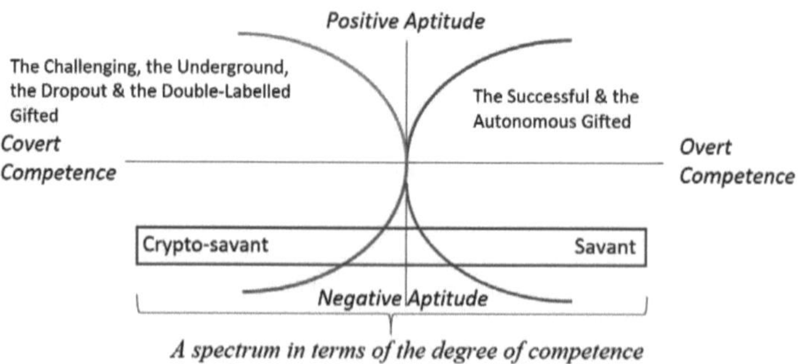

Figure 19. Aptitude-Competence Model of Savantism and Giftedness

Clark (2001) views autistic savants as 'the underserved minority of gifted children with disabilities that require nurturing to realize their savant skill potential and, as such, trialled an educational curriculum (the Savant Skill Curriculum) using a strengths approach by combining strategies currently employed in the education of gifted children (enrichment, acceleration, and mentorship) with those used in autism education (visual supports and social stories). By focusing on the strengths of these individuals and implementing a differentiated curriculum specifically for autistic savants, results were highly successful in the functional application of savant skills and in improved traits related to autism such as behaviour, social skills, and academic self-esteem. Treffert (2000) also recommends focusing on talent, instead of eliminating the defect, as the most useful approach toward increasing socialization, language and independence of savants. In this way, the special skills of the savant become a useful treatment tool as conduit toward normalization, and nurturing the talent also improves the talent itself.

The Treffertian trait #6 concerns literal, eidetic-like memory with massive capacity in the area of expertise. BK has an excellent eidetic-like memory. For instance, he can recall the exact

---

Type 4-The Dropout Gifted: They feel rejected and are angry with adults and with themselves. They may act depressed and withdrawn or respond defensively. Their interests lie outside the realm of the regular school curriculum and they fail to receive support and affirmation for their talent and interest in these unusual areas.

Type 5-The Double-Labelled Gifted: Also known as twice-exceptional, they are physically or emotionally handicapped in some way, or who have learning disabilities.

Type 6-The Autonomous Gifted: Independent, self-directed, and well-respected, they have learned to use the system to create new opportunities for themselves, i.e., they make the system work for them. Often serve in some leadership capacity within the school or community, they have strong, positive self-concepts because their needs are being met. Being so successful as learners, they receive positive attention and support for their accomplishments as well as for who they are.

route his parents and/or he himself have taken during a long travel even if that happened for one or first time, and he knows when a wrong turn is made. Although the current IQ test could not assess or confirm his eidetic-like memory because he cannot understand the oral instruction, based on several observations (not only his mother, but others, too) of his travels in foreign countries, BK's memory has a massive capacity in the area of his interest (e.g., what he saw and he could remember all the routes he took to travel to a specific location even he had been there once).

Core Symptom of Over-excitability in One/More Areas of Extreme Interests

The core symptom of over-excitability (see Chia & Lim, 2017, for detail) consists of two Treffertian traits #4 and 5, i.e., obsessive preoccupation with the skill and in BK's case, his skill is painting, and a prolific output of product (i.e., paintings) on a continuous basis, respectively.

Regarding the Treffertian trait #4, BK's skill in painting is not the same as very specific skill (e.g., BK has an obsessive habit of picking up tiny circular items found on the ground anywhere) which may not seem to be related to what the savant is known for (e.g., acrylic paintings done by BK). However, it can be regarded as an essential pre-skill that is very much required in being observant for fine details in drawing or painting. Here are five general skills very important to drawing or painting:

- *Motor control:*

Feeling comfortable with a drawing tool in the hand is important to the drawer. For example, in pen drawings one important element or aspect is having confident and smooth lines. This is much easier with good motor control.

- *A good visual eye:*

Most of the time, many arts teachers have taken this skill for granted. In general, an autistic individual has always been a very visual person. S/he may stare into the leaves of the trees and appreciates the colour, texture, and unique qualities of each individual leaf. S/he may stare into the clouds and look at the interesting textures and colours the sky makes. S/he may look out the window on car rides and get lost into the world of his/her own even passing by of houses. What does this have to do with drawing? It is having this visual appreciation that has helped the drawer to come up with creative, visual ideas to draw. It also helps the drawer with some layout ideas on the paper and further appreciate the art he/she is creating. For example, BK drew and painted the winter scene. He chose to draw the bare tree on the left side of the paper, not the centre or the right. That means he has some layout idea about his painting.

- *Creativity:*

Creativity is difficult to be measured. It actually depends on the type of art BK is interested in. Creativity is not necessarily required for art, such as in realistic pieces such as still lives. But in general, creativity is very important and necessary in drawing. It is the foundation to the message being communicated, and what makes a piece interesting to look at. It is particularly a creative outlet if it is the sole or primary means with which one communicates. BK in his own way has spoken his voice through his painting and indicates his "sedentary" (spending time being alone or inactive) state of mind as manifested in his latest winter painting.

Treffert discusses the notion of creativity among autistic savant artists. He explains that most begin their artistic careers with striking replicas of what they have seen and stored. However, over time, improvisation begins to appear by omitting an object or inserting one that was not observed in the original image. BK's paintings are replicas of images he and his mother find on the internet. BK indicates which images he likes and wants to paint and that is used as a guide. His paintings have begun to show more interpretation in the recent months, resulting in more personalized results in his paintings. See Figure 20 for the images used as inspiration and the final paintings BK produced as a result. Eventually, interpretation, free form style, or some other form of creativity is expressed in fresh, original work (Hosseini, 2012). See Figure 21 for free form paintings as BK's original work.

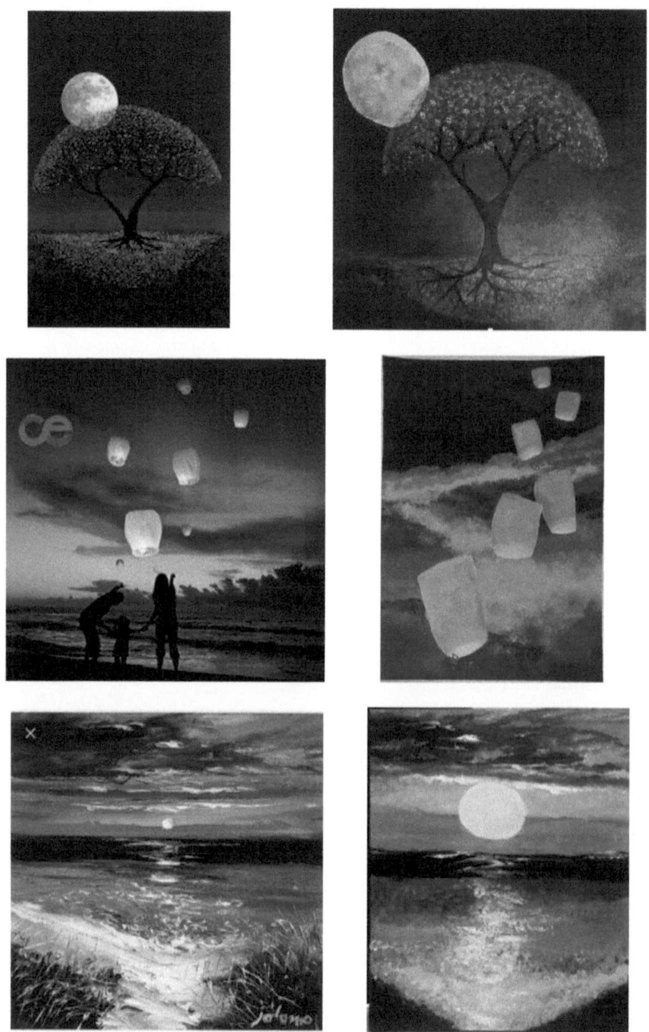

Figure 20. BK's Paintings (right) Interpreted from Images (left) Found on the Internet

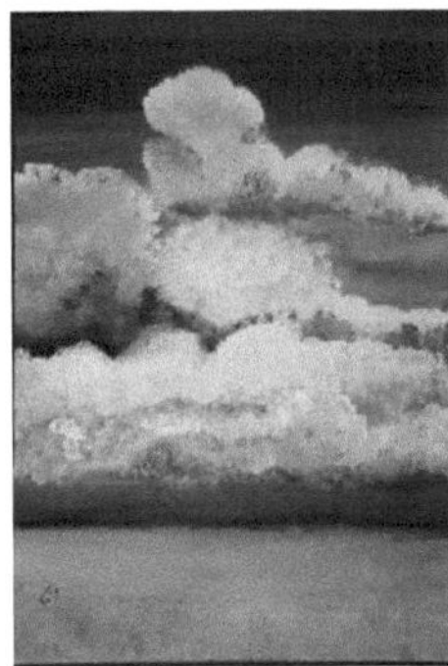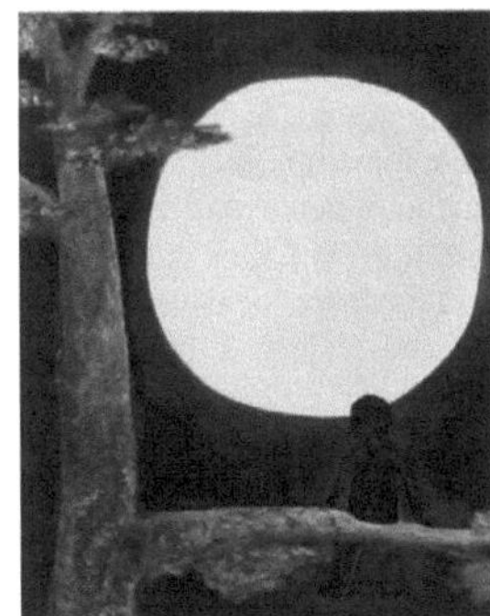

Figure 21. BK's Free Form Paintings

- *Patience:*

The most important skill is patience. Being able to sit down for hours on one piece is very hard. Especially when it is not coming out the way a typical individual wants it to. Patience is required to create a good art piece. Impatience leads to a rushed unfinished job, and overall bad drawing. BK is full of patience and can go on for many hours to do his painting.

- *Tenacity:*

Practice is the most important element to getting better at anything, especially drawing. When drawing, the only way to improve is to draw all the time and keep practicing. Drawing and painting skills, even by the best and most renown artists, takes continuous practice. This is also true of savant artists. It is a natural course of practicing one's craft. Eventually, with enough practice, and dedication, one will see improvement. BK has spent hours, sometimes days, working on the same painting. Typically, an individual with severe disability would get bored very quickly or easily and never stay on-task for even a few minutes. Yet BK perseveres. He is making progress over time with some facilitation, guidance and support provided to him. Anybody with normal intellectual capacity will also make progress over time with and without facilitation, guidance and support. We do not see it as something "not right" to facilitate, guide and support a savant or crypto-savant artist especially if he/she has other handicapping condition that is interfering with the painting/drawing ability. This has to do with the degree of assistive support that is required so that the drawer can proceed with his/her drawing/painting with least disruption resulted from his/her current condition. This is termed this as Universal Design for Learning and its seven principles serve to help and not restrict someone with special needs like BK to do what he/she loves to do, i.e., painting.

BK also displays another type of tenacity when it comes to subject matter for his paintings. As seen in Figures 5 and 6, the moon is the main subject in each painting. He tends to fixate on a particular subject as the central theme for his painting and will persist in that subject matter until he indicates he has done enough and will express a new interest. In four months, BK produced seven new paintings all centred around the moon theme, initially inspired by seeing a news cast on television about the blood moon. He has since moved on to beach and clouds as the central theme to his paintings.

Finally, the Treffertian trait #5 of a prolific output of product on a continuous basis is noted in BK's production of his paintings over a period of time. Frequency will depend on his readiness and mood to do so just like a typical artist will draw or paint when there is inspiration. This is also dependent, however, on his access to materials. Since BK has very limited communication, he may not always be able to communicate his desire effectively to paint or describe the materials he needs and wants to produce a new work. For a long time, BK's parents have not understood or recognized his talent and did little to foster it. Only more recently have they begun to facilitate his access to materials to paint more frequently. BK now paints regularly, two to three sessions per week. Each session lasts approximately 2 hours. He produces usually two, sometimes three, completed paintings per month. Given his difficulties and the coordination required by his mother to facilitate painting sessions, this is a remarkable result.

The re-conceptualizing of autistic savantism as a spectrum syndromic disorder (ASSSD) reflects the complex presence of symptoms that often accompany such a diagnosis. The insertion of *spectrum* in the label is a reminder that the presentation of talent or skill (or disability) varies within the general clinical population, as a continuum into the general population, and between the subgroups within the clinical population, as described earlier and no two autistic savant artists will progress in the same manner. This reframing of the distinguishing features that characterize a savant artist (i.e., core symptoms: underlying disability, over-excitability in one or more areas of extreme interest, and underlying superior systemizing abilities) includes the understanding that many autistic savants have co-morbid disorders that disrupt the artistic process in ways that are different to the autistic savants who do not.

BK's case has served to explore the operating definition of savant syndrome and consider other perspectives and conceptualizations of this rare condition. As more cases, like BK's, are examined and analysed against the defining characteristics of autistic savant or savant syndrome, and now autistic savant spectrum syndromic disorder, we broaden and advance our understanding of the manifest symptoms that hallmark this rare and enigmatic condition.

CHAPTER FIVE
CONCLUDING REMARK

As reported by Camulli, Goh and Chia (2018), "BK's earlier diagnosis done at a public hospital in Singapore showed that he has Tuberous Sclerosis Complex (TSC) – an autosomal dominant disorder resulting from mutations in the TSC1 or TSC2 gene" (p.121). Epilepsy is present in 70%-90% of individuals with TSC and often develop within the first year of life. Developmental and behavioural disorders including autism spectrum conditions (ASC) or autism spectrum disorders (ASD), are also frequently diagnosed in TSC.

According to research studies (e.g., de Vries, Hunt, & Bolton, 2007; Numis et al., 2011; Wong, 2006), ASC affects between 17% and 63% of individuals with TSC, a prevalence dramatically higher than that of the general population. Mental retardation and early onset of epilepsy in TSC, in particular infantile spasms, are associated with the development of ASC/ASD in such individuals. In addition, there is evidence of an association between temporal lobe epileptiform foci with ASC/ASD in TSC.

As a follow-up to the current assessment done, these results will be reviewed in the context of other available information and the current operating definition of savant syndrome. According to Treffert (2010), "[S]avant [S]yndrome is a rare, but extraordinary, condition in which persons with serious mental disabilities, including autistic disorder, have some 'island of genius' that stands in marked, incongruous contrast to overall handicap" (p. 1). Based on this definition, Camulli et al. (2018) safely confirmed that "BK displays signs of Savant Syndrome in the area of art due to his extensive 'literal memory' capacity that exists with this skill of painting" (p.121). "Compared to other artists, a number of distinguishing features characterize the savant artist: underlying disability; innate ability without teaching or training; talent which typically 'explodes' on the scene at a very early age; obsessive preoccupation with the skill; prolific output of product on a continuous basis; and literal, eidetic-like memory with massive capacity in the area of expertise" (Treffert, 2010, p. 21).

ACKNOWLEDGEMENT

The authors wish to thank the parents of BK for their kind agreement to participate in this case study and also for the permission to use the assessment results in the publication of this monograph for the purpose of professional sharing.

REFERENCES

[1] Amberger, J.S., Bocchini, C.A., Scott, A.F., & Hamosh, A. (2019). OMIM.org: Leveraging knowledge across phenotype-gene relationships. *Nucleic Acids Research, 8*(47), D1038-D1043

[2] Asano, E., Chugani, D.C., Muzik, O., Shen, C., Juhasz, C., & Janisse, J. (2000). Multimodality imaging for improved detection of epileptogenic foci in tuberous sclerosis complex. *Journal of Neurology, 54*(10), 1976-1984.

[3] Baron-Cohen, S. (2006). Autism: The empathizing-systemizing (E-S) theory. The year in cognitive neuroscience. *Annals of the New York Academy of Sciences, 1156*(1), 68-80.

[4] Baron-Cohen, S., Ashwin, E., Ashwin, C., Tavassoli, T., & Chakrabarti, B. (2009). Talent in autism: Hyper-systemizing, hyper-attention to detail and sensory hypersensitivity. *Philosophical Transactions of the Royal Society, 364*(1522), 1377-1383.

[5] Baron-Cohen, S., Richler, J., Bisarya, D., Gurunathan, N., & Wheelwright, S. (2003). The Systemising Quotient (SQ): An investigation of adults with Asperger syndrome or high functioning autism and normal sex differences. *Philosophical Transactions of the Royal Society, Series B, Special issue on "Autism: Mind and Brain", 358*, 361–374.

[6] Baron-Cohen, S., & Wheelwright, S. (2004). The empathy quotient: An investigation of adults with Asperger syndrome or high functioning autism, and normal sex differences. *Journal of Autism and Developmental Disorders, 34*(2), 163-175.

[7] Beery, K.E. (1997). *The Beery-Buktenica VMI: Developmental test of visual-motor integration with supplemental developmental tests of visual perception and motor coordination: Administration, scoring, and teaching manual* (4th ed.). Parsippany, NJ: Modern Curriculum.

[8] Bleuler, E. (1911). *Dementia Praecox oder Gruppe der Schizophrenien*. Leipzig, Germany: Deuticke.

[9] Bleuler, E. (1978). *Dementia Praecox or the Group of Schizophrenias* (Monograph Series on Schizophrenia No. 1.) (9th Imprint). New York: International Universities Press.

[10] Bozzao, A., Manenti, G., & Curatolo, P. (2003). Neuroimaging. In P. Curatolo (Ed.), *Tuberous sclerosis complex: From basic science to clinical phenotypes* (pp.109-123). London, UK: Mac Keith Press for the International Child Neurology Association.

[11] Brown, L., Sherbenou, R. J., & Johnsen, S. K. (1997). *TONI-3, test of nonverbal intelligence: A language-free measure of cognitive ability*. Austin, TX: Pro-ed.

[12] Camulli, E.J., & Goh, L.A.L. (2018). Re-conceptualizing autistic savantism as a spectrum syndromic disorder: A sequel to the case study of a young adult savant artist. *European Journal of Special Education Research, 3*(4), 185-204.

[13] Camulli, E.J., Goh, L.A.L., & Chia, K.H. (2018). A case study of a young adult savant artist with tuberous sclerosis complex. *European Journal of Special Education Research, 3*(2), 109-124.

[14] Carsillo, T., Astrinidis, A., & Henske, E.P. (2000). Mutations in the tuberous sclerosis complex gene TSC2 are a cause of sporadic pulmonary lymphangioleiomyomatosis. *Proceedings of the National Academy of Sciences, 97*(11), 6085-6090.

[15] Chia, K.H. (2007 April). How God spoke to me through one child with autism. *Faithlink*, 98-100.

[16] Chia, K.H. (2008a). Two case studies of autistic savants: Understanding their systemizing ability (Paper #101-4.4). Paper presented at the 10th Asia-Pacific Conference on Giftedness: Nurturing talents for the global community, Hong Kong Association for Gifted Education. Retrieved [online], 12 February, 2018, from: http://hkage.org.hk/en/events/080714%20APCG/04-%20Social%20&%20Emotional%20Development/4.4%20Chia_Two%20Case%20Studies%20of%20Autistic%20Savants-%20Understanding.pdf

[17] Chia, K.H. (2008b). Autistic savant: A need to re-define autism spectrum disorder (ASD) (Paper No.1). In *Special educational needs series* (pp.1-17). Singapore: Cobee Publishing House.

[18] Chia, K.H. (2008c). Newsbites: Math patterns. *Autism-Asperger's Digest, Fall(4)*, 33.

[19] Chia, K.H. (2008d). How I taught one high-functioning autistic child to perform multiplication. *The Educational Therapist, 29*(2), 22-24.

[20] Chia, K.H. (2012). Autism enigma: The need to include savant and crypto-savant in the current definition. *Academic Research International, 2*(2), 234-240.

[21] Chia, K.H., & Camulli, J.E. (2017). A proposed symptomatological-nosological classification system for learning and behavioral disruptions: What educational therapists should know from disabilities/disorders per se to multiplex disabilities/disorders. *European Journal of Special Education Research, 2*(6), 124-145.

[22] Chia, K.H., & Lim, B.H. (2017). Understanding overexcitabilities of people with exceptional abilities within the framework of cognition-conation-affect-and-sensation. *European Journal of Education Studies, 3*(6), 649-672.

[23] Chorianopoulos, D., & Stratakos, G. (2008). Lymphangioleiomyomatosis and tuberous sclerosis complex. *Lung, 86*(4), 197-207.

[24] Clark, T.R. (2001). The application of savant and splinter skills in the autistic population through curriculum design; a longitudinal multiple-replication case study. Unpublished PhD thesis, University of New South Wales, Australia.

[25] Clarke, A., Hancock, E., Kingswood, C., & Osborne, J. P. (1999). End-stage renal failure in adults with the tuberous sclerosis complex. *Nephrology, dialysis, transplantation: Official publication of the European Dialysis and Transplant Association-European Renal Association, 14*(4), 988-991.

[26] Cooijmans, P. (2003). IQ and real-life functioning. Retrieved [online] from: https://paulcooijmans.com/intelligence/iq_ranges.html.

[27] Crino, P.B., Nathanson, K.L., & Henske, E.P. (2006). The tuberous sclerosis complex. *New England Journal of Medicine. 355*(13), 1345–56.

[28] Dabrowski, K. (1972). *Psychoneurosis is not an illness*. London, UK: Gryf.

[29] de Vries P.J., Hunt, A., & Bolton, P.F. (2007). The psychopathologies of children and adolescents with tuberous sclerosis complex (TSC): A postal survey of UK families. *European Journal of Child and Adolescent Psychiatry, 16*, 16–24.

[30] Deweerdt, S. (2014). Distinct features signal autism risk in tuberous sclerosis. Retrieved [online] from: https://www.spectrumnews.org/news/distinct-features-signal-autism-risk-in-tuberous-sclerosis/.

[31] DiMario, F.J. (2004). Brain abnormalities in tuberous sclerosis complex. *Journal of Child Neurology, 19*(9), 650-657.

[32] DiMario, F.J. Jr., Sahin, M., Ebrahimi-Fakhari, D. (2015). Tuberous sclerosis complex. *Pediatric Clinics of North America, 62*(3), 633–648.

[33] DSM History. (April 4, 2018). Retrieved [online] from: https://www.psychiatry.org/psychiatrists/practice/dsm/history-of-the-dsm

[34] Dunn, W. (1999). *Sensory profile: User's manual*. San Antonio, TX: Psychological Corporation.

[35] Exkorn, K. (2005). *The autism sourcebook; Everything you need to know about diagnosis, treatment, coping, and healing*. New York, NY: Regan Books.

[36] Flanagan, D.P., & McGrew, K.S. (1997). A cross-battery approach to assessing and interpreting cognitive abilities: Narrowing the gap between practice and cognitive science. In D.P.

Flanagan, J.L. Genshaft, & P.L. Harrison (Eds.), *Contemporary intellectual assessment: Theories, tests, and issues* (pp.314-325). New York: Guilford Press.

[37] Gallagher, A., Grant, E.P., Madan, N., Jarrett, D.Y., Lyczkowski, D.A., & Thiele, E.A. (2010). MRI findings reveal three different types of tubers in patients with tuberous sclerosis complex. *Journal of Neurology, 257*(8): 1373-1381.

[38] Gibbs, V., Aldridge, F., Chandler, F., Witzlsperger, E., & Smith, K. (2012). Brief report: and exploratory study comparing diagnostic outcomes for autism spectrum disorders under DSM-IV-TR with the proposed DSM-5 revision. *Journal of Autism and Developmental Disorders, 42(8),* 1750-1756.

[39] Gillberg, C., & Coleman, M. (1996). Autism and medical disorders: A review of the literature. *Developmental Medicine and Child Neurology, 38*(3), 191-202.

[40] Gilliam, J.E. (1995). *Gilliam autism rating scale (GARS): Examiner's manual.* Austin, TX: Pro-Ed.

[41] Goh, L.A.K, & Xie, G.H. (2019). A case review of a male Chinese savant adult with tuberous sclerosis complex and syndromic low-functioning/non-verbal autism. *Research in Social Sciences, 2*(1), 13-28.

[42] Gomez, M.R. (1987). Tuberous sclerosis. In M.R. Gomez (Ed.), *Neurocutaneous diseases. A practical approach* (pp.30-52). Boston, MA: Butterworths.

[43] Goncharova, E.A., & Krymskaya, V.P. (2008). Pulmonary lymphangioleiomyomatosis (LAM): Progress and current challenges. *Journal of Cell Biochemistry, 103*(2), 369-382.

[44] Griffiths, P.D., Bolton, P., & Verity, C. (1998). White matter abnormalities in tuberous sclerosis complex. *Acta Radiologica, 39*(5), 482-486.

[45] Guo, X., Tu, W.J., & Shi, X.D. (2012). Tuberous sclerosis complex in autism. *Iran Journal of Pediatrics, 22*(3), 408-411.

[46] Hermelin, B. (2002). *Bright splinters of the mind: A personal story of research with autistic savants.* London, UK: Jessica Kingsley.

[47] Holland, B.A., Kucharczyk, W., Brant-Zawadzki, M., Norman, D., Haas, D.K., & Harper, P.S. (1985). MR imaging of calcified intracranial lesions. *Radiology, 157*(2), 353-356.

[48] Hosseini, D. (2012). *The art of autism: Shifting perceptions.* San Diego, CA: Art of Autism Publisher.

[49] Howlin, P., Goode, S., & Hutton, J. (2009). Savant skills in autism: Psychometric approaches and parental reports. *Philosophical Transactions of the Royal Society B: Biological Sciences, 364,* 1359-1368.

[50] Huang, J., & Manning, B.D. (2008). The TSC1-TSC2 complex: A molecular switchboard controlling cell growth. *Biochemistry Journal, 412*(2), 179-190.

[51] Huerta, M., Bishop, S.L., Duncan, A., Hus, V., & Lord, C. (2012). Application of DSM-5 criteria for autism spectrum disorder to three samples of children with DSM-IV diagnoses of pervasive development disorders. *American Journal of Psychiatry, 169*(10), 1056-1064.

[52] Hurley, R.S., Losh, M., Parlier, M., Reznick, J.S., & Piven, J. (2007). The broad autism phenotype questionnaire. *Journal of Autism and Developmental Disorders, 37*(9), 1679-1690.

[53] Jeste, S.S., Hirsch, S., Vogel-Farley, V., Norona, A., Navalta, M.C., Gregas, M.C., Prabhu, S.P., Sahin, M., & Nelson-III, C.A. (2013). Atypical face processing in children with tuberous sclerosis complex. *Journal of Child Neurology, 28*(12), 1569-1576.

[54] Jeste, S.S., Wu, J.Y., Senturk, D., Varcin, K., Ko, J., McCarthy, B., Shimizu, C., Dies, K., Vogel-Farley, V., Sahin, M., & Nelson-III, C.A. (2014). Early developmental trajectories associated with ASD in infants with tuberous sclerosis complex. *Neurology, 83*(2), 160-168.

[55] Kandel, J. (2016). What skills are required for drawing? Retrieved [online] from: https://www.quora.com/What-skills-are-required-for-drawing.

[56] Kellogg, R. (1970). *Analyzing children's art*. Mountain View, CA: Mayfield Publishing.

[57] Knowles, M.A., Habuchi, T., Kennedy, W., & Cuthbert-Heavens, D. (2003). Mutation spectrum of the 9q34 tuberous sclerosis gene TSC1 in transitional cell carcinoma of the bladder. *Cancer Research, 63*(22), 7652-7656.

[58] Kraepelin, E. (1887a). *Die Richtungen der psychiatrischen Forschung: Vortrag, gehalten bei der Übernahme des Lehramtesan der kaiserlichen Universität Dorpat*. Leipzig, Germany: Vogel.

[59] Kraepelin, E. (1887b). *Psychiatrie: Ein kurzes Lehrbuch für Studirende und Aerzte (2nd ed)*. Leipzig, Germany: Abel.

[60] Krause, L. (2019). Syringomyelia. Retrieved [online] from: https://www.healthline.com/health/syringomyelia.

[61] Lai, M-C., Lombardo, M.V., Chakrabarti, B., & Baron-Cohen, S. (2013). Subgrouping the autism spectrum: Reflections on DSM-5. *PLoS Biology, 11(4)*, 1-7.

[62] Landa, R.J., Gross, A.L., Stuart, E.A., & Bauman, M. (2012). Latent class analysis of early developmental trajectory in baby siblings of children with autism. *Journal of Child Psychology and Psychiatry, 53*(9), 986-996.

[63] Lewis, W.W., Sahin, M., Scherrer, B., Peters, J.M., Suarez, R.O., Vogel-Farley, V.K., Jeste, S.S., Gregas, M.C., Prabhu, S.P., Nelson-III, C.A., & Warfield, S.K. (2013). Impaired language pathways in tuberous sclerosis complex patients with autism spectrum disorders. *Cerebral Cortex, 23*(7), 1526-1532.

[64] Lim, B.H., & Chia, K.H. (2017). A psycho-educational evaluation and profiling of a male crypto-savant with non-verbal low-functioning autism. *International Journal of Multidisciplinary Research and Development, 4*(6), 396-410.

[65] Melillo, R. (2012). *Autism: The scientific truth about preventing, diagnosing, and treating autism spectrum disorders and what parents can do now*. New York: A Penguin Group.

[66] Meyers, C.E., Nihira, K., & Zetlin, A. (1979). The measurement of adaptive behavior. In N.R. Ellis (Ed.), *Handbook of mental deficiency, psychological theory, and research (2nd ed.)* (pp.70-91). Hillsdale, NJ: Erlbaum.

[67] Miller, L.K. (1999). The savant syndrome: Intellectual impairment and exceptional skill. *Psychological Bulletin, 125*(1), 31–46.

[68] Mohkam, M., Shohadaii, S., Kompani, F., Aghadoost, H.R., Seyed, A.H.S.A., & Nasrin, E.N. (2014). Tuberous sclerosis presenting with acute kidney failure, pyelonephritis, and polycystic kidney disease. *Iranian Journal of Kidney Disease, 8*(4), 336-340.

[69] Moolten, S.E. (1942). Hamartial nature of tuberous sclerosis complex and its bearings on the tumor problem: Report of a case with tumor anomaly of the kidney and adenoma sebaceum. *Archives of Internal Medicine, 69*(4), 589-623.

[70] Moritz, K.P. (Ed.) (1783-1793). *Gnothi Sauton oder Magazin der Erfahrungsseelenkunde als ein Lesebuch fur Gelehrte and Ungelehrte. Vol. I-X*. Berlin: August Mylius: 1783-1793.

[71] Myers, P., Baron-Cohen, S., & Wheelwright, S. (2004). *An exact mind: An artist with Asperger syndrome*. London, UK: Jessica Kingsley Publishers.

[72] National Institute of Neurological Disorders and Stroke (NINDS) (2006, April 11). *Tuberous sclerosis fact sheet*. NIH Publication No. 07-1846. Retrieved [online], 3 January, 2018, from: https://www.ninds.nih.gov/Disorders/Patient-Caregiver-Education/Fact-Sheets/Tuberous-Sclerosis-Fact-Sheet.

[73] Nie, D., Di Nardo, A., & Han, J.M. (2010). TSC2-RHEB signaling regulates EphA-mediated axon guidance. *National Neuroscience, 13*(2), 163-172.

[74] Northrup, H., Koenig, M.K., Pearson, D.A., & Au, K.S. (1999). Tuberous Sclerosis Complex. In M. P. Adam, H.H. Ardinger, R.A. Pagon et al. (Eds.), *GeneReviews® [Internet]* (pp.1993-2019). Seattle, W.A.: University of Washington. Retrieved [online] from: https://www.ncbi.nlm.nih.gov/books/NBK1220/.

[75] Numis, A.L., Major, P., Montenegro, M. A., Muzykewicz, D. A., Pulsifer, M. B., & Thiele, E. A. (2011). Identification of risk factors for autism spectrum disorders in tuberous sclerosis complex. *Neurology, 76*, 981-987.

[76] Oot, R. F., New, P. F. J., Pile-Spellman, J., Rosen, B. R., Shoukimas, G. M., & Davis, K. R. (1986). The detection of intracranial calcifications by MR. *American Journal of Neuroradiology, 7*, 801-809.

[77] Pierangelo, R., & Giuliani, G. (2006). *The special educator's comprehensive guide to 301 diagnostic tests*. San Francisco, CA: Jossey-Bass.

[78] Prather, P., & de Vries, P. J. (2004). Behavioural and cognitive aspects of tuberous sclerosis complex. *Journal of Child Neurology, 19,* 666-674.

[79] Regier, D. A., Kuhl, E. A., & Kupfer, D. J. (2013). The DSM-5: Classification and criteria changes. *World Psychiatry, 12*(2), 92-98.

[80] Reynolds, C.R., & Hickman, J.A. (2004). *Draw-a-person intellectual ability test for children, adolescents, and adults*. Austin, TX: Pro-Ed Inc.

[81] Ridler, K., Suckling, J., Higgins, N., Bolton, P., & Bullmore, E. (2004). Standardized whole brain mapping of tubers and subependymal nodules in tuberous sclerosis complex. *Journal of Child Neurology, 19*(9): 658-665.

[82] Ridler, K., Suckling, J., Higgins, N. J., de Vries, P. J., Stephenson, C. M., Bolton, P. F., & Bullmore, E.T. (2007). Neuroanatomical correlates of memory deficits in tuberous sclerosis complex. *Cerebral. Cortex, 17*(2), 261–71.

[83] Roach, E.S., & Sparagana, S.P. (2004). Diagnosis of tuberous sclerosis complex. *Journal of Child Neurology, 19*(9): 643-649.

[84] Roid, G.H. (2003a). *Stanford-Binet intelligence scales-5th edition (SB-5)*. Itasca, IL: Riverside Publishing.

[85] Roid, G.H. (2003b). *Stanford-Binet intelligence scales-5th edition: Examiner's manual*. Itasca, IL: Riverside Publishing.

[86] Roid, G.H., & Barram, R.A. (2004). *Essentials of Stanford-Binet intelligence scales (SB5) assessment*. Hoboken, NJ: John Wiley & Sons.

[87] Roid, G., Miller, L., Pomplun, M., & Koch, C. (1997). *Leiter international performance scale-revised (LIPS-R)*. Wood Dale, IL: Stoelting Co.

[88] Sampson, J.R. (2003). TSC1 and TSC2: Genes that are mutated in the human genetic disorder tuberous sclerosis. *Biochemical Society Transactions, 31*(3): 592-596.

[89] Sasson, N.J., Lam, K.S., Childress, D., Parlier, M., Daniels, J.L., & Piven, J. (2013). The broad autism phenotype questionnaire: prevalence and diagnostic classification. *Autism Research, 6*(2), 134-143.

[90] Saulnier, C.A., & Klaiman, C. (2018). *Essentials of adaptive behavior assessment of neurodevelopmental disorders*. Hoboken, NJ: John Wiley & Sons.

[91] Schopler, E., Reichler, R., & Renner, B.R. (1988). *The childhood autism rating scale*. Los Angeles, CA: Western Psychological Services.

[92] Shields, W.D. (2006). Infantile spasms: Little seizures, big consequences. *Epilepsy Currents*, *6*(3), 63-69.

[93] Şıklar, Z., & Berberoğlu, M. (2014). *Syndromic disorders with short stature. Journal of Clinical Research in Pediatric Endocrinology, 6*(1),1-8

[94] Simons, B.J. (2004). *Seven steps to a successful painting.* Canada: The Author (Self-Published).

[95] Siroky, B.J., Yin, H., & Bissler, J.J. (2010). Clinical and molecular insights into tuberous sclerosis complex renal disease. *Pediatric Nephrology, 467,* 1689-1695.

[96] Sparrow, S.S., Balla, D.A., & Cicchetti, D.V. (1984). *Vineland adaptive behavior scales-interview edition: Survey form manual.* Circle Pines, MN: American Guidance Service.

[97] Sparrow, S.S., Cicchetti, D.V., & Balla, D.A. (2005). *Vineland adaptive behavior scales-2nd edition (VABS-2).* Circle Pines, MN: American Guidance Service.

[98] Staley, B.A., Montenegro, M.A., Major, P., Muzykewicz, D.., Halpern, E.F., Kopp, C.M., Newberry, P., & Thiele, E.A. (2008). Self-injurious behaviour and tuberous sclerosis complex: Frequency and possible associations in a population of 257 patients. *Epilepsy & Behaviour. 13*(4), 650-653.

[99] Treffert, D.A. (2000). Savant syndrome. In Kazdin A.E. (Ed.), *Encyclopedia of psychology,* Volume 7 (pp. 144-148). Washington, DC: American Psychological Association.

[100] Treffert, D.A. (2009). The savant syndrome: An extraordinary condition. A synopsis: past, present, future. *Philosophical Transactions of the Royal Society B: Biological Sciences, 364* (1522): 1351-1357.

[101] Treffert, D.A., (2010). *Islands of genius: The bountiful mind of the autistic, acquired, and sudden savant.* London, UK: Jessica Kingsley Publishers.

[102] Treffert, D.A. (2010). *Extraordinary people: Understanding savant syndrome.* New York, NY: Ballantine Books.

[103] Treffert, D.A. (2014). Savant syndrome: Realities, myths and misconceptions. *Journal of Autism and Developmental Disorders, 44,* 564-571.

[104] Tuberous Sclerosis Association, (2017a). *Tuberous sclerosis complex and the heart.* London, UK: The Author.

[105] Tuberous Sclerosis Association, (2017b). *An introduction to tuberous sclerosis complex.* London, UK: The Author.

[106] Umeoka, S., Koyama, T., Miki, Y., Akai, M., Tsutsui, K., & Togashi, K. (2008). Pictorial review of tuberous sclerosis in various organ. *Radio Graphics, 28*(7): e32. Available from: https://pubs.rsna.org/doi/pdf/10.1148/rg.e32.

[107] U.S. National Library of Medicine, (2019). Tuberous sclerosis complex. Genetic home reference. Available from: https://ghr.nlm.nih.gov/condition/tuberous-sclerosis-complex#genes.

[108] Wechsler, D. (1997). *Wechsler Adult Intelligence Scale-3rd Edition (WAIS-3).* New York: Pearson Education.

[109] Wheelwright, S., Baron-Cohen, S., Goldenfeld, N., Delaney, J., Fine, D., Smith, R., Weil, L., & Wakabayashi, A. (2006). Predicting autism spectrum quotient (AQ) from the systemizing quotient-revised (SQ-R) and empathy quotient (EQ). *Brain Research, 1079*(1), 47-56.

[110] Whitney, R.V. (2016). *Definitions of sensory terms.* Retrieved [online], 26 February, 2018, from: http://www.spdbayarea.org/definition_of_sensory_terms.htm.

[111] Wilson, C., Idziaszczyk, S., Parry, L., Guy, C., Griffiths, D.F., Lazda, E., Bayne, R.A., Smith, A.J., Sampson, J.R., & Cheadle, J.P. (2005). A mouse model of tuberous sclerosis 1

showing background specific early post-natal mortality and metastatic renal cell carcinoma. *Human Molecular Genetics, 14*(13): 1839-1850.

[112] Wong, V. (2006). Study of the relationship between tuberous sclerosis complex and autistic disorder. *Journal of Child Neurology, 21*, 199–204.

Content:

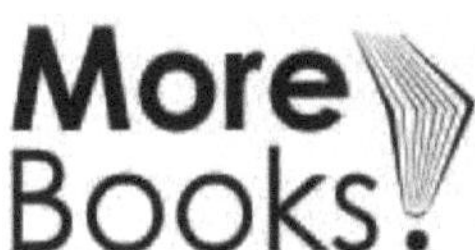

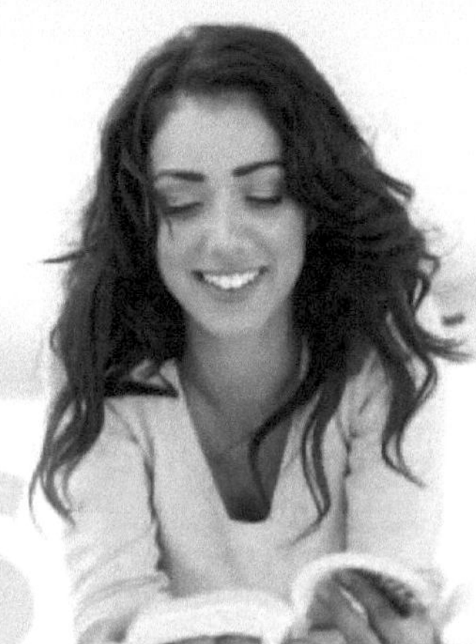

Buy your books fast and straightforward online - at one of world's fastest growing online book stores! Environmentally sound due to Print-on-Demand technologies.

Buy your books online at
www.morebooks.shop

Kaufen Sie Ihre Bücher schnell und unkompliziert online – auf einer der am schnellsten wachsenden Buchhandelsplattformen weltweit! Dank Print-On-Demand umwelt- und ressourcenschonend produziert.

Bücher schneller online kaufen
www.morebooks.shop

KS OmniScriptum Publishing
Brivibas gatve 197
LV-1039 Riga, Latvia
Telefax: +371 686 204 55

info@omniscriptum.com
www.omniscriptum.com

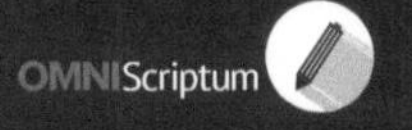

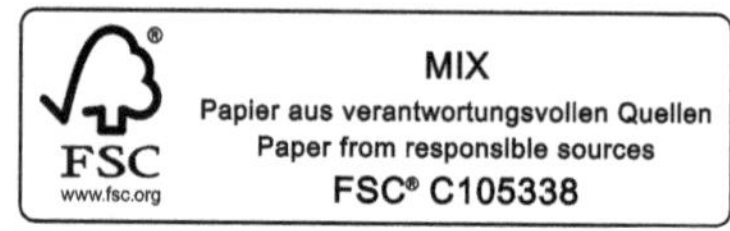

Printed by Books on Demand GmbH, Norderstedt / Germany